MW00787952

Advanced Praise for
A Fullness of Uncertain Significance

In this tender and candid collection of short essays, Dr. Bruce Campbell illuminates how much medicine is truly the sacred act of holding vigil with and for our patients. Through his reflections, we get a glimpse of how surgeons hone their instincts, grow through challenges, and cope with disappointment as they navigate the uncertainty inherent in medicine. Through his polished lens, the reader understands how even in the pressurized world of surgery, heavy with the responsibility of healing through a scalpel's cuts, there are moments of intimacy that are filled with grace.

—Rana Awdish, MD, FCCP, FACP, author of *In Shock: My Journey from Death to Recovery and the Redemptive Power of Hope*

Dr. Bruce Campbell turns his scalpel on his own history as a surgeon, probing the medical field past, present, and future. His vibrant stories illuminate the fundamental human underpinnings of medical science, bringing to light the glories, tragedies, imperfections, and uncertainties we must all grapple with. Eminently readable and richly satisfying.

—Danielle Ofri, MD, PhD, Clinical Professor of Medicine at New York University School of Medicine, Editor-in-Chief of *Bellevue Literary Review*, and author of *When We Do Harm: A Doctor Confronts Medical Error*

Dr. Campbell's reflections will resonate with those who treat cancer patients as well as those who have had cancer themselves. Medical students and residents will also be inspired by his life's journey as a surgeon and teacher, aspiring to their own joyful and meaningful lives in medicine.

—Julie Ann Freischlag, MD, FACS, FRCSEd(Hon), DFSVS, CEO Wake Forest Baptist Health, CAO Atrium Health, Dean of the Wake Forest School of Medicine, and 2021-2022 President of the American College of Surgeons.

In this rich collection of stories and essays, Dr. Campbell reflects on his years of caring for patients and training young doctors to follow in his footsteps. With compassion, humility, and shimmering prose, he shares the joys, pains, and somber responsibility of being a surgeon.

—Gayle Woodson, MD, surgeon, educator, and award-winning author of *After Kilimanjaro* and *Leaving La Jolla*

Bruce Campbell is no average surgeon and no ordinary writer. He takes the excellence of his medical trade and weaves the challenges, exhilarations, and tough decisions of surgery into beautiful prose. Here is one who clearly doesn't reduce patients to a diagnosis, but who sees them as whole persons worth getting to know. The chapters in this book are like windows into the humility and generosity of a man I'd like to have as my personal physician.

—Peter W. Marty, editor/publisher of *The Christian Century*

With his willingness to delve beneath the surface, Bruce Campbell has created a deftly interwoven series of lessons gleaned from poignant moments of a fulfilling surgical career. In a warm, compassionate, and honest voice, Dr. Campbell delivers to the reader not just insights on medicine, but truths about humanity.

—K. Jane Lee, MD, author of *Catastrophic Rupture: A Memoir of Healing*

Humorous and humble, serious and sublime, these lean essays offer a glimpse behind the surgical drape to show what it's like to be a cancer surgeon over the course of a long, rewarding career. From Campbell's first invitation into the "inner sanctorum" of the O.R. as a nurse's aide while in college, through tender interactions with patients, to his projections about the profession when he is long gone, this smart, sensitive surgeon illustrates how doctors can listen to, care for, and learn from their patients. He courageously goes to the "hard places" as well as sharing those special moments that make it all worthwhile. Early in the collection, Campbell writes, "Besides being a surgeon, I am also a human being." This beautiful book is about both.

—Kim Suhr, MFA, author of *Nothing to Lose* and Director of Red Oak Writing

In lucid and succinct vignettes, Dr. Campbell illuminates the myriad of emotions and sensations that accompany a life in surgery. These stories of persistence, camaraderie, shame, grief, guilt, and regret are told with a deep humility that springs from a vantage point of experience. These ideas serve as the springboard to discuss unique, personal insights whose wisdom is of import to anyone in the healing profession. With elegant and engaging prose, Campbell beautifully expresses the honor it is to be a physician.

—William Lydiatt, MD, Chief Medical Officer Nebraska Methodist and Women's Hospitals and Professor of Surgery, Creighton University in Omaha, Nebraska

"Over the years, I have made an uneasy truce with failure," says Campbell in the opening pages of his debut anthology, and yet his stories are anything but. Captivating, heart-wrenching, inspiring—he chooses his words as meticulously as he conducts his surgeries.

And it's just like a surgeon to keep you up in the middle of the night. "One more story," you'll tell yourself, but with Campbell's reflections, it's hard to stop. There's a familiar ease with which he flourishes his pen; everything falls away, and it's almost as if you're sitting across the table from him as he recalls. You laugh when he laughs, you cry when he cries, and you wait as he waits. His memoir of stories is sure to become a rite of passage for future doctors and patients alike, enjoyable little tunes that all hum together in a harmony of sound.

Turning the last page of Campbell's novel, I succumb to my own "fullness of uncertain significance"—I have been charged to seek meaning, to reflect, to sit in the silence of his reverberating truths.

—Olivia Davies, MD, poet, writer, and dermatology resident at Massachusetts General Hospital

The words "clarity" and "grace" take on heightened significance in this honest yet lyrical set of essays by Bruce Campbell. The immediacy and intensity of these stories immediately swept me into the consulting room and OR. I felt as if I were a privileged witness to an almost sacred encounter between surgeon and patient. Subtle language lays bare a primal relationship. It is impossible to read this book and not be changed by the experience.

—Carol Scott-Conner, MD, PhD, Professor Emeritus of Surgery at University of Iowa Carver College of Medicine and author of *A Few Small Moments: Short Stories*

Dr. Bruce Campbell sets a new milestone for doctor-writers. As an otolaryngologist and head and neck surgeon, he treats patients with the most advanced and aggressive cancers imaginable. Internists like me wonder how head and neck surgeons like him do it; this book gives me the answer. Dr. Campbell brings luminous sight to his work. His writerly gifts let him capture the delicate and the solemn, the tragic and the everyday dimensions of illness. Not a set of doctorly instructions (though instruct it does), *A Fullness of Uncertain Significance: Stories of Surgery, Clarity, & Grace* lays open the profound mysteries and truths and awe about this life of ours. These stories will change lives.

—Rita Charon, MD, PhD; Bernard Schoenberg Professor of Social Medicine and Professor of Medicine; Chair of the Department of Medical Humanities and Ethics; Executive Director of Columbia Narrative Medicine, Columbia University, New York City; Co-author, *Principles and Practice of Narrative Medicine*

In this compelling, insightful, and beautifully written compendium of stories, Bruce Campbell shares the lessons he has learned, and continues to learn, throughout his medical education and his years as a highly successful surgeon, faculty member, and teacher. *A Fullness of Uncertain Significance* is refreshingly honest and introspective, exploring not only many of the desirable outcomes when he had been faced with a broad array of professional challenges, some potentially life-and-death, but also those outcomes that were less than he had hoped for. Readers will appreciate the author's willingness to reveal that, "As a surgeon, I have made mistakes that have hurt people. This should not surprise anyone since, besides being a surgeon, I also am a human being." Providers, teachers, and students of health care in every field and at every level of service will benefit greatly from what the author has accurately labeled "Stories of Surgery, Clarity, & Grace." This isn't merely a book about one man's life as a surgeon. It is a book about the need for understanding and compassion when dealing with others, especially those in distress.

—Myles Hopper, PhD, JD, author of *My Father's Shadow*

In this collection of essays, Dr. Campbell pulls the reader into his Milwaukee otolaryngology clinic, the operating room, and his medical work in Kenya. He tells story after story with wonder, humour, and affection. He looks back on his medical training and fantasizes about medicine in the mid-twenty-first century. He lets us in on his unique vantage point on humanity, and does so with such humility and grace that his own humanity is never in question.

—Martina Scholtens, MD, author of Your Heart is the Size of Your Fist

A Fullness
of
Uncertain
Significance

———————

Stories of Surgery,
Clarity, & Grace

———————

Bruce H. Campbell, MD FACS

Ten|16
P R E S S

www.ten16press.com - Waukesha, WI

To Kathi

Table of Contents

Try to be one of those people on whom nothing is lost.

- Henry James

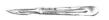

Introduction

It is the 1990s and my new patient, Todd, reminds me too much of myself. Like me, he is in his thirties and has young kids in grade school, a sweet wife, and a modest home a couple of miles from the hospital. He takes care of himself and is faithful with his diet and exercise routines. Todd and Linda spend as much time in the Wisconsin Northwoods as possible and head to national parks every summer. At every visit, they always ask about my family and how I am doing. His parents and friends are supportive and involved. He is at the point in his life when things are finally falling into place.

Until they fall apart.

Todd should never have developed a tongue cancer but, as he acknowledges, "Stuff happens." Fortunately, the mass is small. I take him to the operating room and remove it completely. He is going to be just fine.

Until he isn't.

A few months later, the cancer inexplicably roars back. Big, bleeding tumor. Lots of pain. Metastatic neck nodes overflowing with cancer. He can only eat soup and soft foods.

"Can you fix this?" Todd asks me. "I don't want to die."

I am worried. "I will do everything possible," I reply. And I mean it.

Over the next few weeks, I take him back to surgery and

perform an extensive procedure, concentrating as hard as I possibly can to make certain I remove every last bit of the cancer. The next day, I get on the phone with colleagues around the country to pick their brains. I work with my colleagues at home to coordinate his care. I spend extra time during his appointments as I watch Todd suffer through radiation therapy. I know his cancer is aggressive but am absolutely certain, deep down, that if I pay fastidious, unwavering attention to every detail and obsess over ensuring that everything is done according to protocol, Todd will beat this thing.

It works. For a while.

And then, it doesn't.

More cancer and then more chemotherapy. More tests. More treatment. Even more tests.

Then, not much left to offer.

"I am so tired," he says.

"I am *so* sorry," I tell him.

As he weakens, it becomes too difficult to bring him back and forth to the hospital for appointments. One day, when he is receiving hospice care and is close to death, I call Linda and ask if I can stop by the house. Todd and Linda's home care team has set up his bed in the living room of their bungalow, where he can see out the window to the quiet street, keep an eye on the bird feeders, talk to friends, watch baseball on television, and sit with his kids. Family photos, children's projects, medical supplies, and the accumulated detritus of a life nearing its premature end are everywhere.

I step around a coffee table laden with hospital bills. He brightens as I come across the room and grip his hand. My stomach is in knots. "Good to see you," I say. The fetor of his rotting tumor hangs in the air. To me, it is the smell of failure. He has a tracheotomy and can no longer speak. "Thanks for coming," he mouths then closes his eyes. Linda pulls the blanket up over his shoulders.

I stay for a few minutes. I talk to Linda and tell his mother how much knowing him means to me. They show me a few photographs of Todd before he was sick. I say goodbye and walk back to my car, realizing I will never see him alive again.

What did I do wrong? I tried everything I could think of, brought to bear every strategy, made every phone call, worked with every consultant, explored every option, and still. And still. Todd reminds me of myself. I weep when he dies.

Over the years, I have made an uneasy truce with failure, yet my mind and my heart still view each other warily. I understand that the statistical probability of Todd's survival was determined much more by cancer biology and the intricate interplay of genetics and immunity than it was by what I brought to bear as a surgeon. My heart tells me, though, that it was my responsibility – and within my grasp – to beat the odds, to overcome the laws of nature, to overwhelm molecular mysteries that have yet to be unlocked, to work a miracle.

When a radiologist pauses to scrutinize an inexplicable finding on a CT scan, she spends time trying to decide what it represents. If, despite her best efforts manipulating and reformatting the images, the mysterious shadow fails to reveal its secret, she might dictate that the area contains "a fullness of uncertain significance." The "fullness" might go on to represent the first sign of recurrent cancer, a smoldering infection, or a finding of no consequence whatsoever. Later, when I read her report, it becomes my responsibility to discern what the fullness most likely represents. Is it a harbinger of danger or something we can watch for a while? I commit to accompany the patient until the dilemma has been completely explored.

Over the months, Todd had many scans and X-rays that included the equivalent of "a fullness of uncertain significance." Each time, we sorted through the possibilities. If I could explain the fullness and it did not represent anything worrisome, we did nothing. If the cause was unclear, though, we decided whether to do an additional test, order a biopsy, or possibly repeat the scan in a few weeks or months. In every case, though, the "fullness of uncertain significance" initiated a conversation, some reflection, and a shared decision.

Over the course of my career, many patients and families have shared their histories and experiences which revealed unexpected or surprising insights. These stories usually flew past me, but more than a few made me stop and think, *Huh? Really?* These glimpses became, to me, the narrative equivalent of the "fullness of uncertain significance" I had seen on X-rays and scans. As with the clinical "fullnesses," these narrative "fullnesses" compelled me to stop in my tracks and offer my full attention until I had wrestled with what they might mean. At times, I explored these fragments of insight by writing down what happened, what I heard, or what surprised me. By committing some of these experiences to words, I represented the lessons I hoped I would never forget. A few grew into the essays in this collection.

The process of haphazardly pouring words onto a page – and then sorting through them to make some sense of things – has enriched my life and helped me come to terms with the uncertainty inherent in my career that mixes surgery, cancer care, teaching, and research. This includes the experiences that have brought both distress and joy. I am still discovering that I deserved no more undue praise for miraculous moments than I deserved all of the blame for bleak times of bitter disappointment.

The stories in this book – including my emotions and reactions – are real, although nonessential details have been rearranged and names changed in the interest of HIPAA-compliance. In many instances, as I sought to make sense of encounters, I created essays "in the shadow" of events, writing a few hours or days after they occurred. In other instances, it took decades until I was finally ready to commit a story to words.

A life in medicine, particularly during training and early practice, consists of an endless maelstrom of chaotic and overwhelming experiences pulling young physicians down dark and lonely tunnels. These can be dangerous, fraught places. For me, turning these ambiguous emotions and experiences into narratives offered a respite as I struggled to come to terms with my own imperfections and humanity. In this book, I share a bit of what emerged when I slowed down and realized what my patients, families, and colleagues – people like Todd and Linda – were showing me as I attempted to haltingly accompany them on their difficult and unknowable paths.

The relationships with my patients offered me moments of clarity and grace. I am honored to share these stories with you.

PART ONE

The Road to Becoming a Surgeon

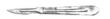

Inner Sanctum

You cannot connect the dots looking forward;
you can only connect them looking backwards.
- Steve Jobs

"Doesn't that window open any wider? Bring in another fan!" the surgeon demands.

It is summer in Chicago in the early 1970s, and air conditioning won't be installed in the hospital for a few more years. Beads of sweat gather at the edge of the orthopedic surgeon's cloth cap, and he calls the circulating nurse to step up periodically to wipe his forehead. Heat and city noise roll through the open windows and into the operating room. The brief morning rain shower has left the shiny, green floor nearest the windows glistening and wet. Even from the seventh-floor operating room, the staff can hear the sounds of people talking and laughing at the bus stop in front of the hospital. Diesel fumes from the bus occasionally waft through the screens. A car honks on the boulevard. Pigeons land on the sill and peer in.

"Sorry, Doctor. We don't have any more fans."

He scowls. "Can you at least get me a cup of sterile ice water?"

I am home from college on break and working as a nursing assistant in a hospital near where I grew up. In an arrangement that I suspect would be impossible a few decades later, they hire me back whenever I return home for a few days. I plan to apply to medical school during my senior year in college and view opportunities to work in a hospital as a kind of rehearsal. It is a chance that I try very, very hard not to take for granted.

For this particular school break, I am assigned to the OR where I clean rooms, restock supplies, transport patients, set up cases, fold linens, make coffee, run errands, track down X-rays, mop hallways, scrub bathrooms, and do whatever else is needed. Occasionally, when one of the OR staff members is at lunch, I am pressed into duty as a completely unqualified surgical assistant.

Today, the charge nurse tells me to scrub into the orthopedic case so one of the other nurses can go on break. I carefully scrub my hands and forearms as I have been taught, put on a gown, and step up to the table. The surgeon looks at me. "Remind me your name again, son . . . Bruce? Okay, here, Bruce," he says. "Hold her leg steady. I need to fix the hip fracture, and it will go a lot more smoothly if all of the parts don't move." He is a folksy, hardworking character.

He grips my hand and wrist and shows me exactly how he wants things to line up. He sets to work.

These are the days before CT scans and prefabricated femoral prostheses. The repair will be based on the physical exam, a couple of plain X-rays, and the surgeon's ingenuity. The doctor learned many of his trauma skills as a military surgeon in Vietnam and is accustomed to figuring out how to best use the available metal plates, screws, wires, pins, and plaster. He drills the holes with a power drill like the one my dad keeps on his workbench in the garage.

"Back when I was in school, these sorts of fractures were treated with casts, traction, and bed rest," he tells me. "These days, we fix 'em."

I surmise that this isn't an easy break to repair. I want to help but know nothing about hip fractures. I hold still as best I can. Eventually, I begin to sense his rhythm. Things move along, and I get the hang of how he wants the leg stabilized. Soon, he is humming an aria as he lines up the fragments. "There you go!" he says to me. "That went well. You did a fine job holding still, son. She's good as new."

Those early experiences remain fresh. I remember the layout of many of the ORs where I worked over the decades. I can conjure up the hum of the old Bovie electrosurgical machines and feel the conductive grounding strips tucked inside my shoes – a throwback to the era before mine when static electricity could lead to an explosion of volatile anesthetic agents like cyclopropane and ether. I can remember listening to the voice of the hospital operator over the hallway speakers in the days before pagers and text messaging. I remember the surgeons who inspired me and scared me as I contemplated a surgical career. And, I am grateful to the cranky otolaryngologist who pointed me toward my life's calling.

The nurse returns from her break, and I scrub out. I watch the surgeon sew up the incision and place the dressings. After he leaves, I help move the patient onto a cart and then wheel her to the recovery room. Before long, I am back in the same OR, holding a mop handle instead of the patient's leg, but also knowing that I am one step closer to what I want to do with my life.

The Fifth of July

*It is extraordinary what a difference there is between
understanding a thing and knowing it by experience.*
- St. Teresa of Avila

"I'm so sorry! Tell my mom I'm so sorry!"

I hear him before I see or smell him. Ten-year-old Scott is sobbing and apologizing as the ambulance cot rolls down the ramp from the parking area and into the small emergency room where I am working as a nursing assistant during a summer break from college. The driver and attendant cradle him in a sheet and lift him onto the open cart. I help get him positioned on the bed and get a whiff of his clothes. It is the first time I inhale the unforgettable combination of burnt cotton, gunpowder, and singed flesh.

It is the fifth of July. Back in those days, all sorts of fireworks were still allowed within city limits. When I was younger, I, too, had been one of the kids who looked forward to Independence Day by accumulating sparklers, poppers, caps, bottle rockets, snakes, and paper packs of Black Cat firecrackers – anything that involved smoke, fire, or noise. We had envied the big kids who could afford more firepower, as they set off M-80s, cherry bombs, and entire packs of the firecrackers.

As little kids, my friends and I broke apart packs of firecrackers, untangling the fuses and pulling them out of the packages one by one. On a dare, someone held onto a single lit firecracker for as long as he dared, tossing it in a dangerously random direction just before the fuse burned down to nothing. More than occasionally, someone waited too long and was rewarded with ringing ears and buzzing fingertips. It was, of course, a completely stupid thing to do. We all thought it was absolutely hilarious.

On this particular fifth of July, we piece together Scott's story.

Earlier this morning, he and some of his friends went to the city park near his home where, last night, a group of older kids had set off hundreds of bottle rockets and strings of firecrackers. It was clear and dry overnight and, as the boys had walked around the park, they gathered together a treasure trove of duds – the intact firecrackers that no longer had fuses. They found the metal pipe the older boys used last night to launch bottle rockets. *How cool!* they must have thought. *We can send a shower of flame way up in the sky!* They likely pictured an amazing, canon-like display of pyrotechnics. Someone found some leftover safety matches and a piece of newspaper. The show was about to begin.

Somehow, Scott was chosen to perform the actual firing of the canon. He carefully jammed the newspaper into one end of the pipe and then dropped all the loose firecrackers into the other. He likely had tried to steady the pipe on the ground or against a tree trunk, but I imagine it kept falling over. Finally, to steady the pipe in the only way he could think of, he sat down, rested his back against a tree, and held the pipe securely between his legs. He aimed the pipe into the air while one of his friends lit the paper.

I can only imagine the boys' excitement as they waited for the flame to catch and work through the paper. Did they wonder if the pipe might get too hot to hold? Had Scott adjusted the angle to avoid hitting the other kids? Did anyone have second thoughts? I don't think to ask.

Although Scott must not have had time to admire the blast, it was probably very impressive. The flame reached the dry firecrackers. The explosives obeyed the laws of physics as they ignited, sending hot gas, smoke, and flaming debris out both ends of the pipe simultaneously. His shorts caught fire. His friends took off running as fast as they could.

A neighbor heard the explosion and saw what had happened. Soon, Scott is on the stretcher in the emergency room.

His shorts are cut off and his wounds inspected. The doctor finds that Scott has a superficial, but extremely tender, burn very high up on both of his thighs. The results of the blast are not pretty, but everything is intact. It could have been much worse.

His mother soon arrives and takes a look at his injury. She shakes her head. "Scott, sweetie, what were you thinking?"

Scott does not answer. The emergency room nurse shows Scott's mother how to clean the burn and apply salve. She tucks the prescription for the cream into her purse and promises to make a follow-up appointment with the pediatrician. She hands Scott an undamaged pair of shorts from home. "We'll step out now, and you can get dressed."

We hear him slowly slide off the cart and can see his feet below the curtain. He gingerly pulls up his pants. "Mom, this hurts!"

"That's too bad, sweetie," she replies. "We'll pick up more of the burn cream on the way home." She smiles at the nurses. "Just remember, Scott, some of life's lessons hurt more than others."

The rings on the ceiling track rattle as the curtain is pulled back, revealing the boy, legs held slightly apart, standing next to the cart and staring at the floor. Scott holds his mother's hand as he hobbles gingerly out the door and up the ramp toward the parking area. I return to the cubicle to make the bed, straighten up the supplies, and empty the trash. The space still smells of burnt cotton and gunpowder, but the smell of singed flesh has already begun to fade.

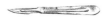

Problem Solved

The best cure for insomnia is to get a lot of sleep.
- WC Fields

Early one morning, during a summer when I am working as a nursing assistant, one of the surgeons drops by our emergency room in a particularly good mood. The emergency room physician, who is between patients, asks him why he is so happy.

"It was the first night in a week that I did not get a 2:30 a.m. phone call from Mrs. Swanson," he replies. I pretend to work but keep listening.

"Really? Why does she call you at night?"

"Well, it seems that since being discharged from the hospital after surgery, she hasn't been sleeping well at all. I prescribed medication, relaxation, exercise, dietary change . . . anything I could think of . . . but she could not sleep! She was spending hours each night roaming throughout her house."

"And . . . ?"

"And so, when she couldn't sleep, she would call me at my house at 2:30 a.m. and tell me how miserable she was! Every night, the phone would ring and there she would be!"

"What would she say?"

"Not much. Same thing every night. 'Doctor, are you asleep? I can't sleep, Doctor! Can't you give me something? I feel so tired, Doctor! When will I sleep?' I was running out of ideas."

The emergency room doctor wrinkles his forehead. "Why didn't you tell her to call in the morning?"

"I *did* tell her that, of course. It just didn't make any difference."

They stand silently for a while. I'm not certain what the surgeon is thinking, but I'm certain the ER physician is trying to come up with other treatment options. The absurdity of the situation percolates for a few moments; I think we are all picturing the bleary-eyed woman forlornly padding around in a robe and slippers, repeatedly checking the clock, and finally picking up the phone to make her nightly call. "It was ridiculous," says the surgeon. "I imagined it going on forever."

The other physician holds up his hand. "But, wait! You said you slept through the night last night . . ."

"No, I didn't say that. What I said was, 'I didn't get a call at 2:30 a.m.' . . ."

The physician scratches his head. "What do you mean?"

"I mean she didn't call *me*."

"Oh, no! What?! You didn't . . ."

"Of course, I did! At 3:00 a.m., my alarm went off. I picked up the phone and called *her*! 'Were you sleeping, Mrs. Swanson? You were? Oh, that's wonderful! I'm so happy for you! I just wanted to make sure you were doing okay! Uninterrupted sleep is so refreshing, don't you think? Well, good night!' She mumbled something in return. I'm pretty confident that will be our last middle-of-the-night conversation!"

The ER physician shakes his head. The surgeon grins and pushes the metal plate on the wall, and the doors slide apart. He is humming as he heads down the corridor towards the elevator that will take him to the operating room where he will find his first patient of the day, IV started and medications ready, all set to be put to sleep.

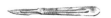

The Hidden Curriculum

*Students undergo a conversion in the third year of
medical school: not "preclinical" to "clinical,"
but "pre-cynical" to "cynical."*
- Abraham Verghese, MD

It is a Saturday morning in the minor procedure clinic next
to the emergency room. I am a first-year medical student and still
working at the hospital as a nursing assistant. A crusty surgeon
calls to tell us that he will be meeting a woman with a perirectal
abscess in our clinic in a few minutes and to have everything set
up. I collect the supplies, prepare the local anesthetic, show the
woman where to change her clothes, and wait while she puts on
a hospital gown. She is very uncomfortable and refuses the offer
of a chair. We wait for the surgeon to arrive.

The surgeon breezes in and grunts at us before rinsing his
hands and pulling on a gown and gloves. "Lie on your side
facing away from me," he barks. "Tuck your knees up as high
as you can!" He scoffs as he places the sterile drapes around her
rectum. "Higher! I gotta see this thing." He looks at me. "Hand
me that local." He injects some of the anesthesia into the skin
overlying and around the infected abscess. The patient squirms.
"Hold still, dammit!"

I have never seen a perirectal abscess but can tell that the patient is miserable. The surgeon picks up the scalpel and presses it into the abscess a couple of times, looking for the softest area of the swollen, red, and inflamed mass that peeks through the opening in the sterile drapes. The patient clutches the stiff emergency room pillow against her face, moaning as she rocks back and forth. Whenever the surgeon manipulates the abscess, she yelps.

The surgeon sits on a rolling exam chair next to the patient's bed and peers at me over his mask. "You have two jobs: hold her in a position so I can get to her rectum, and then get a culture of the contents once I open this thing up." I nod.

The surgeon holds his gloved hands at the ready and speaks distinctly to the back of the patient's head. "Okay," he says, "you might feel some pressure." I adjust the exam light, then hold the culture swab at the ready. He presses the mass again and then plunges the blade deep inside.

During a recent medical school microbiology lecture on bacteria that thrive in oxygen-poor environments, I learned that they have a distinct odor and that samples of pus must be placed into the culture media quickly. Without knowing it, I am about to confirm those lessons and learn several more.

As the abscess opens, pus flies out, releasing an overpowering stench worse than anything I could ever have expected. I recoil as gray-brown pus as thick as heavy cream pours through the drapes, cascades down onto the table, then spreads out on the sheet. My eyes burn as the surgeon glances at me with, what I assume is, amusement. "Here," he points. "Get the culture now." I sweep up some of the fluid with the swab and push it onto the culture tube. The surgeon presses on the abscess with his thumbs to evacuate as much pus as possible, tapes on a dressing, and pulls off his gloves. He writes a quick note in her chart then hands me the paperwork. "Tell her to call the office for an appointment next week." He wheels and heads out the door.

Serendipitous, formative, and important moments are common to all medical students and physicians, yet because of their spontaneity, they are not part of any written curriculum. Over the years, I learned many lessons in the clinic, at the bedside, and in the operating room that I would have learned in no other way except by having been present when they happened.

The day I watched the incision and drainage of the perirectal abscess in the clinic, I realized for the first time that pus in an abscess cavity can exist under pressure. I learned that it is possible for a person to scream in pain and then say, "Thank you! *Oh, thank you!*" with the same breath. I developed an indelible association between a mixed bacterial abscess and the word "putrid." And it would take me years to unlearn that when a surgeon notices a student's distress, it is apparently just fine to smirk, say nothing, and go on your way.

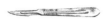

Harbinger

The outline of your future path already exists,
for you created its pattern by your past.
- Sai Baba

My girlfriend, Kathi, has planned a home-cooked steak dinner to celebrate the six-month anniversary of our first date. This is no simple task, since she lives in a tiny campus apartment that consists of a closet, a bed, a desk, and a sink. There is no kitchen on her floor. She plans to stage the meal preparation by first warming the vegetables and then broiling the steaks in her toaster oven. We already bought what we needed for a lettuce salad and picked out an affordable bottle of wine that we will drink from glasses borrowed from the hospital cafeteria. On the day of the dinner, she borrows a candle from a friend and claims one of the two shared common rooms down the hall. We look forward to our evening together.

We are both students. Kathi is completing her nursing degree, and I am in my fourth year of medical school. I am working less and less at my job as a nursing assistant because of my schedule. We live in neighboring buildings on the medical center campus on Chicago's Near West Side.

On our special day, I am on the Medicine Service, an

overwhelmingly busy rotation where there is never enough time to finish all of the work or reading. I am awake every third night on call. Despite it all, I am learning a lot and am impressed with the residents to whom I have been assigned, especially Tom, the chief resident who runs our team. He is smart, capable, and unflappable in a crisis. I want to learn as much as possible from him during my rotation. Thanks, in part, to his influence, I am strongly considering choosing Internal Medicine as my future specialty.

Around lunchtime, I run into Kathi in one of the hospital wards. "Things aren't too busy today. We only have a couple of planned admissions," I tell her. "I should be able to get to your place by 5:30." Her apartment is right across the street from the hospital's main entrance.

"Okay," she says. "Give me about a fifteen-minute warning, so I can get the steaks started."

The afternoon drags by as I think about our dinner plans. I check labs, run down reports, order X-rays, and write notes in patient charts. I have learned the survival lessons that all students must master while adjusting to eighty-to-hundred-hour workweeks. As my final assignment of the day, I admit a man who has come into his doctor's office with worsening diabetes and gout. I write out his history and physical, work with the team to complete his orders, and make a list of things that the overnight on-call student will track down. Finally, I am done.

I pick up the phone outside the conference room and call Kathi. "I'm grabbing my coat and heading out," I say while checking the clock. It is just 5:30. "Sorry I didn't get there on time. I'll be there by 5:45. 6:00 at the latest."

"Perfect," she says. "I figured you would be a couple of minutes late. The veggies are warm. I'll put the steaks on, so they'll be ready."

As I hang up the phone, a nurse bolts out of the room across the hall. "Mr. Riley just collapsed!" she shouts. "I can't find a pulse. Call a code!"

The floor jumps into action. Tom and the junior residents, who are finishing up their daily charting in the conference room next door, rush across the hall and into Mr. Riley's room. I drop my coat and follow. The overhead speaker system announces, "CODE BLUE! TWO PAVILION! ROOM 27!" and the corridor is quickly jammed with nurses, respiratory therapists, doctors, and support staff arriving from around the hospital. I am swept into the room and stand at the periphery of the crowd, trying to see what is happening. I figure I can watch for a few minutes and then head out.

The code cart is wrestled into a spot next to the bed. One of the nurses grabs a clipboard from the cart and begins charting everything that happens. The patient in the other bed in Room 27 looks horrified. Someone pulls the curtain between the beds, although it doesn't hide much.

Tom's eyes narrow as he scans the room and initiates the code protocol. He leans over the bed. "Mr. Riley!" he yells next to the dying man's ear. "Can you hear me?" No response. "Okay, start compressions. Hook up the EKG!"

One of the residents begins CPR. The EKG machine sits on top of the code cart and two people attach its cables with elastic straps to Mr. Riley's arms and legs. In the 1980s, EKG machines spew yards of paper strips which soon cover the floor around the cart. The compressions stop for a few seconds while an anesthesiologist inserts an endotracheal tube. "Tube's in!" she announces. She tapes the tube to his face and attaches and rhythmically squeezes the breathing bag. Someone listens to the lungs with a stethoscope. "Bilateral breath sounds!" The compressions resume.

"Check for pulses." Mr. Riley is a big man, and he bounces up and down in the bed as the compressions continue. His face, which had been purple when we rushed into his room, is beginning to show some pink again. One of the nurses feels for the artery in his groin. "I can feel the femoral," she says. "Feels strong." The room is packed.

The team soon locks into a cadence of chest compressions and breaths. Just as I slide a step toward the door, Tom points at me. "Bruce, take over on compressions." I move into position, lock my fingers together, and rhythmically press Mr. Riley's sternum halfway to his spine, pausing whenever the anesthesiologist squeezes the oxygen bag. This is something I have done in the emergency room and am comfortable with the process. It makes me feel as though I am helping. After several minutes, one of the residents takes my place and I fade to the back of the room, realizing I am late for dinner yet hoping I will get to help again.

Lab tests return. "Show me the labs. He's acidotic," says Tom. "Give him an amp of bicarb. He needs potassium, too!" More tubes of blood head to the lab. More IVs, more meds, more labs. Mr. Riley isn't getting better, but he isn't getting worse, either. I take another turn doing chest compressions. I move closer to Tom, trying to imagine what he is thinking with each new lab result and anticipating each medication choice. He is playing chess with death.

After several more minutes, Tom announces, "Okay, hold the compressions. Let's take a look at the rhythm again." The compressions stop, and several people crowd around the EKG machine to stare at the paper strip. "Well, he has a rhythm now, but he's in sinus brady," announces one of the residents. "He's at about twenty per minute. Definitely sinus, though."

"He came in with bradycardia yesterday, but his only symptom was being a bit tired," says a resident, looking through his chart. "He was scheduled to get a pacemaker tomorrow."

"Shoulda had it yesterday. Okay, resume compressions. Let's give him 0.5 milligrams of atropine," said Tom. "Draw up another milligram and tell me when five minutes have passed. And get some epinephrine ready. We'll probably need a drip. Is there a transcutaneous pacer on the code cart?"

One of the nurses yanks open the drawer. "No pacer."

Tom looks around the room. "Bruce, go up to the ICU and grab one of the pacers. Don't forget the wires! Someone call ahead and let them know Student Doctor Campbell will be coming to pick it up."

"Okay. On my way." I bolt from the room, full of purpose once again. Our ward is on the second floor, and the ICU is on the ninth. The elevators are impossibly slow this time of day. *It will be quicker to take the stairs,* I think. I veer into the stairwell and climb all the way, two steps at a time. *Don't waste a step,* I think to myself. Despite being in the hospital for hours on end, I rarely feel as though I am actually contributing something useful or making a difference in the lives of the people I encounter. This, somehow, feels different. I hope that the pacer might give Mr. Riley a chance.

I emerge on the ninth floor and trot down the hallway to

the ICU where one of the nurses is expecting me. "Here you go," she says, "and here are the leads. And bring it back if you don't use it."

I turn to go. "Thanks," I say. I run into a housekeeping cart.

"Careful!" calls the nurse. "Don't get overheated."

"Yeah, sure. Thanks." I glance down at my blue, button-down Oxford shirt and tan khaki pants – the unofficial uniform of the 1970s male medical student. My sprint up the stairs has left me drenched in sweat. I wipe my hands on my short white coat, grab the doorknob of the stairwell, and head back down to the second floor as quickly as I can. When I emerge, I run down the hall to Mr. Riley's room. "Tom, here's the pacer!" I call out.

The chest compressions have stopped. "Good. Thanks. Hold onto it for now. The epi got his rate up a bit. He's making a comeback." Tom looks at an EKG strip and glances up at me. He smirks. "Took the stairs, eh?" He counts out the boxes on the EKG. "Okay, his rate's been steady around 60. Does he have a pressure?"

"Around 100 palpable."

"Okay," says Tom. "Let's pack him up and move him to the ICU. When did he get his last dose of bicarb?"

The nurse recording the medications checks her notes and looks up. "7:15."

"Okay, it's been a while. Draw up another syringe and give it. Bring some epi along on the trip to the ICU, as well. Bruce, give me the pacer and I'll return it. You're not on call, right? You take off."

"No. Not on call. Thanks."

The entourage pushes the bed, all of the IV poles, and Mr. Riley out the door and heads down the hallway toward the elevator. The floor is covered with pieces of paper, plastic bags, streaks of blood, IV tubing, and a haphazard pile of EKG strips. It is quiet. The patient in the other bed peeks at me around the curtain. "He gonna be okay?"

"I don't know. I hope so."

I look at my watch. It is 7:40. I am seriously late.

I grab my stuff and head down the hallway, down a flight of stairs, through the lobby, across the street, and up the elevator to Kathi's floor.

I am still trying to air out my shirt when I arrive. "Hi, sweetie," I say. Kathi looks up but says nothing. She sits at the table with a half-empty glass of wine. The vegetables are cold and brown. The steaks are dry and inedible.

"I am so sorry," I say. "There was a code on our floor." My mind runs through a list of explanations. *I couldn't get to a phone. A man's life was in the balance, and they needed me. It was an emergency. I learned a lot. Tom asked me to help. This is what I am preparing to do with my life.* I look at her and realize that it is best to stay silent.

Kathi looks me in the eye. "This meal was important to me, and I believed you when you said you were coming. I'm sure there were plenty of people there to help, right?"

"I am so sorry."

We eat the salads in silence. That evening forty years ago remains fresh.

I don't remember whether Mr. Riley recovered or if he finally got a pacemaker. I do remember, though, how Tom stayed calm in the midst of chaos and managed to teach me about EKGs, resuscitation management, and acute cardiac decompensation. I remember the feeling that I was helping when I ran back from the ICU even though the transcutaneous pacemaker wasn't needed.

And I remember how my excitement was overwhelmed by a wave of regret as I walked in the door and saw the look on Kathi's face.

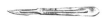

The Procession

Can anybody remember when the times were
not hard and money not scarce?
- Ralph Waldo Emerson

During my senior year in medical school, our entourage trails the snowy-haired professor in and out of the rooms lining the long hospital corridor. Between two doorways, he brings our column to a halt and then grills us all about the patient whose bedside we have just left. "What was he hiding?" "How did he smell?" "What did you notice on his bedside table?" "Describe his fingernails!" He shifts back and forth on his wing tips, the crease of his lab coat sleeves sharp, his bow tie impeccably rendered. When he looks up again, his expression reflects both our lack of observational prowess and the enormous gaps in our knowledge. We proceed down the hall, vowing to be more observant. We know, however, that we will never, ever live up to his expectations.

Just before entering the next room, he turns to face us again, slowly and pointedly speaking to the youngest members of our group.

"Ladies and gentlemen, let me tell you about my first day of internship. We were sitting in the auditorium wearing our short, white jackets and matching hospital-issued pants. I distinctly remember the chairman striding to the lectern. He cleared his throat with great gravitas and scanned our faces. He was clearly not impressed with what he saw. Then the old man pointed his finger at us and announced, 'Gentlemen!' – and we were all men, by the way – 'Gentlemen, there are two things I want you to understand. First of all, do not even *think* about getting married over the coming twelve months! During your time here under my direction, you will rarely leave this very building, and you will be far too busy for such foolishness. This would not be a good time to make such decisions. And secondly, gentlemen, I want you to look to your left and then to right. One of the three of you will have washed out before you finish the coming year. Don't let it be you!' With that, the old man strode out of the room. Our internship was officially underway."

The professor swivels and disappears into the next room, expecting us to follow on his heels. Our jaws go slack. We gloomily fall in line, and I bury my left hand with its shiny new wedding band into the pocket of my rumpled short, white coat.

Many years later, a senior medical student asks about my experiences. "So, exactly how hard was training back when you were a resident?" She has heard that things are different now than they were in the "bad old days," but she remains anxious about what waits for her during her upcoming internship and residency. "You know, back before the eighty-hour workweek?"

What should I tell her? We withstood long hours, had very little supervision, endured abusive surgical personalities, and lived in a "see one, do one, teach one" culture. Residency was more about moving the indigent through clinic than it was about educating a generation of compassionate physicians. But no matter how hard we worked, it was always made abundantly clear that training had been even more difficult for the generation that had preceded us. Chief residents delighted in sharing anecdotes of on-call nights that included *twice* as many patient workups and *half* as much sleep. Call schedules in those days were always more rigorous than ours. Whenever we thought about how badly we wanted to get home, we would hear from an attending physician how he was required to enlist in the Army or Navy Reserve to decrease the possibility of being drafted and ending up as a General Medical Officer in Vietnam. Everyone knew secondhand, cautionary tales of residents being summarily fired for leading an attending into the wrong patient room, accidently bumping a surgeon's shoulder in the OR, or making minor errors in judgment.

Because we had heard so many stories from our seniors, we were convinced that training had become gentler over the years. We believed that we were the recipients of this good fortune and stumbled gratefully through medical school and residency despite miserable stretches of every-other-night call, no semblance of "a weekend," and hours of pointless busywork. We looked forward to our fourteen days of vacation. Classmates at other institutions or in other departments reported less sleep and more abuse. We persevered by knowing that we would eventually graduate.

Residents have always felt like indentured servants. Medical students have forever been anxious about their current challenges and what they will soon face as residents. My young student is no different.

"I mean," she asks, "how did you get through it?"

"Well," I confirm, "it was hard. The hours were often very long."

She frowns.

A host of images appears. The painful stories are replaced by the faces of special patients and fellow trainees from years ago. I hear the distinct but fading voices of long-departed teachers. The oppressive aloneness dissipates as I remember the peals of laughter that accompanied middle-of-the-night practical jokes. I recall specific hospital employees who helped us just because they were decent people. I remember the unearned, grace-filled moments of intimacy with families undergoing the worst kind of stress, and I marvel that we managed to somehow emerge relatively intact from our halting, unaided experiences facing grief and death.

I pause. "But, it wasn't all bad. Here, let me tell you a story one of my professors told me many years ago about *his* training while we were making rounds."

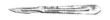

Answering the Question

*Twenty years from now you will be more disappointed
by the things you didn't do than by the ones you did
do. So, throw off the bowlines. Sail away from the
safe harbor. Catch the trade winds in your sails.*

\- Mark Twain

Head and neck cancer surgeons know when "The Question" is coming. A casual conversation eventually turns to, "What do you do for a career?" The pleasant exchange is replaced with talk of disfigurement and life-threatening illness. The person's brow furrows. "How can you deal with that day after day? Isn't it depressing? Why didn't you pick something happier for a career?"

These are legitimate questions. As a medical student many years ago, I enjoyed every rotation and wondered how I would ever narrow down my choices and pick a specialty. Eventually, I decided that I was most content in the operating room. Even when I knew I would become a surgeon, there were still dozens of trajectories which my career might have taken.

It is a spring afternoon in 1980, and I am a twenty-five-year-old senior medical student. I am sitting in a folding chair in a departmental conference room, listening to a visiting out-of-town cancer surgeon. He runs through his slideshow, describing a procedure he devised to restore voice for patients who have undergone removal of their voice boxes. It is a complex operation that involves the creation of tubes of lining tissues that shunt air from the trachea to the back of the throat and then through the mouth, thus allowing the person to speak.

It is an interesting presentation but, at my level of training, I am confused by the approach and the diagrams. I am years away from doing any type of surgery like this on my own. At some point during his talk, I begin to check my watch, wondering when the conference will end.

Then, the visiting surgeon flips the controls and adjusts the volume on a 16mm movie projector. The light flickers as the film moves past the bulb. There, on the screen, is a man who has undergone a total removal of his voice box. The surgeon asks him a question, and the patient responds by holding a vibrating device against his neck to create an artificial, machine-like sound that he shapes into words. He is understandable, but his voice sounds synthetic.

The next scene shows the same patient after he has undergone the voice-restoring procedure. This time, he answers questions by bringing his hand up to his neck and covering his stoma to redirect air from his lungs through the shunt and into his throat. He is able to talk! The sound is natural and fluent.

I am as much enthralled by his ability to speak as by his enormous smile at the end of the movie. Once the presentation is complete, the senior surgeons ask technical questions about the operation and whether it might cause more problems than it solves. I, on the other hand, am amazed. All I can think is, *I want to be able to do something like that!*

Although the procedure described by the visiting surgeon never caught on (there are much simpler techniques today), that movie steered me toward a career devoted to patients with head and neck cancer. I trace the rest of my life to that day. A few weeks later, I was humbled when a cancer patient's family included me in their circle while making difficult end-of-life decisions. That sealed it.

Even today, when someone asks me "The Question" about how I can possibly do what I do for a living, I tell them about the movie that showed how a patient was given back the gift of speech. I tell them how it made me sit up and see, for the first time, what I wanted to do with my life. I still smile when I describe the man's grin.

Often enough, I have been privileged to see my own patients light up. It is, indeed, all worthwhile.

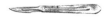

Hearing V. Listening

*The freedom of patient speech is necessary ... [or] ...
the doctor may not be told something vital.*

- Jerome Groopman, MD

One day during my residency in the early 1980s, I am in the ENT Clinic at the Milwaukee County Hospital. I pick up a patient chart from the bin, knock on the old wooden door, and enter the exam room.

My patient looks up and greets me with a smile and a firm handshake. He is a dapper, mustachioed gentleman in his eighties. He has worked for several decades in a large, noisy brewery and lives in one of Milwaukee's ethnic working-class neighborhoods. He returns to the clinic to review his hearing test results. The effects of age and his long-term noise exposure have led to a very severe nerve-deafness.

I start to explain the results of the hearing tests to him.

"You will have to speak much louder, young man!" He is nearly shouting at me to hear his own voice. "I am deaf, you know!"

I start again and review the audiogram with him. I tell him he would benefit from hearing aids.

"Young man, how much would such hearing aids cost, do you think?"

In the 1980s, a set of good hearing aids costs almost $1000. Medicare never has covered the cost, so the expense would be entirely out-of-pocket.

"Oh, Doctor! That is too much! I live on social security and a small pension! How would I ever pay for such a thing?"

It is a serious problem, one that will continue indefinitely. But, in his case, I have an idea. I ask if he was in the military.

"Oh, yes, Doctor! I was in the infantry during The Great War! What an experience that was! We marched clear across Europe!"

His time in the military is good news. Although the rules will change later, I explain that the Department of Veterans Affairs provides hearing aids to all World War I vets regardless of how they lost their hearing. "There will be some paperwork," I tell him, "but you should soon have some help. I know the audiologists at the VA. Hang on a few minutes, and I will help get you information and an appointment to see the hearing aid specialist."

I start writing out the instructions for him on where to go and who to contact. I am pretty proud of myself on this one.

"Doctor . . ."

I keep writing.

"Doctor . . ." He becomes more insistent.

"What is it, Mr. Schmidt?"

"No, Doctor. This won't work, I am quite certain they will not give me the hearing aids at the VA."

"Of course, they will! You served honorably! All World War I vets are eligible for the hearing aids. I know these people, and they will gladly help you."

"No, Doctor, they won't!"

"Why on Earth, not?"

He lets out a belly laugh. "Because, Doctor, during the war, I was on the wrong side!"

I smile and set down my pen. "You are right. That would be a problem." It is so important to listen carefully to the patient's entire story.

Teaching by Example

Whatever we learn to do, we learn by actually doing it;
men come to be builders, for instance, by building,
and harp players by playing the harp.
-Aristotle

I groan. "Don't make me operate with him again! I assisted him in surgery just last week!"

I am the low person on the team, and there is no point arguing. All of the residents and fellows keep track of the rotation and I know it is, indeed, my turn. "What torture!" I whimper as I trudge off to the operating room.

So, why do we all resist working with this particular surgeon? After all, he is a renowned expert with impeccable credentials. He is well-trained and seasoned. He works hard and is never abusive. He always performs unique, inventive procedures, and his approaches are instructive.

The problem: he is hopelessly uninterested in teaching.

One day, for example, I scrub in with him. The patient has large facial cancers and will need extensive removal of skin and major reconstruction. Given the extent of the disease, I know that the case will take several hours to complete.

I arrive in the operating room and introduce myself

although we had met before in conferences. Given his reaction, I suspect he doesn't remember me. "Doctor, I'm Bruce Campbell," I say. "I am one of the new fellows. I look forward to scrubbing with you."

He nods and mumbles, "Hello." That is the last direct verbal interaction between us all day.

The patient is prepared, and the surgery is soon underway. For several hours, I stand across the table from the prominent surgeon and watch. He performs every single maneuver of the procedure from making the first incision to placing the final stitch. When he needs something retracted, he asks the scrub tech to hand him the appropriate instrument. He then places the retractor in the incision and, without looking up, points the back end of it toward me, indicating I am to grab the retractor and pull. If it slips or I try to move it so that it might offer better exposure, he grunts, shakes his head, and moves the instrument back to where it had been.

And so it goes through the entire case. He works through areas with interesting anatomy, none of which he describes. He changes his approach a time or two without revealing his thoughts. He never shares what he is seeing or stops to say, "see how this feels here," or "take the knife and dissect this." He keeps working.

When the case is over, he places the dressings and secures everything with surgical tape. He pulls off his gloves and leaves the room. I stay behind to help transfer the patient to the recovery room and complete all of the postoperative paperwork. I am exhausted.

I realize, of course, that every patient has the right to expect that the senior surgeon will perform their surgery, even in academic teaching hospitals. This expectation is even stronger now than it was during my training.

Yet, the operating room remains a wonderful classroom. It has been so for generations. This is the place where the next cohort of surgeons safely learns what to do and, more importantly, what not to do.

I look back on my experiences with the uninterested teacher with sadness. What more might I have learned? I observed his techniques but never understood why he approached cancers as he did. Now that he is gone, I will never know.

I hope to be remembered as a surgeon who loved to teach, benefiting not only my own patients, but also the patients of my trainees far into the future.

INTERLUDE

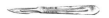

Mom's New Pacemaker

None are so old as those who have outlived enthusiasm.
-Henry David Thoreau

My mother, bless her ninety-year-old heart, is slowing down. The things that made her happiest – getting to church, visiting friends, taking walks, and wandering the aisles in the grocery store – are increasingly difficult. She worries that her lack of energy will soon make every activity impossible.

In 2005, she is living alone in Chicago, about ninety miles from us. My father died suddenly the year before, and she is settling into the life of a widow. She had always been very healthy and upbeat, but she's become more and more fatigued. "What do you think it is?" she asks. "Do you think it is my heart?"

"Let's find out." We arrange an appointment with her internist. Sure enough, her heart rate is uncharacteristically slow and does not speed up when she walks or moves about.

"I believe you need a pacemaker," her doctor confirms. "I'll arrange a visit with a cardiologist."

This gives my mother something new to worry about. "I'm too old for any procedures," she says. "Do you think I could tolerate having a pacemaker?"

We calm her fears as we all wait for the appointment. Within a few days and after a couple of tests, we learn that she might, indeed, benefit from a pacemaker. In a few more days, she is at the hospital and on the schedule. I drive the two hours, pick her up, and help her check in for her procedure.

Everything goes perfectly. The rest of the day, she naps off-and-on. "I'm a little sore," she decides. "You can go home. I'm fine."

"That's okay, Mom," I tell her. "I'll stay with you. You sleep today. Tomorrow, I'll take you home and get you settled."

The next morning, she is alert, sitting up in bed and looking well-rested. Before discharge, she needs a teaching session with the cardiologist's nurse practitioner.

"It's like a little computer that you wear under your skin," the nurse says. She explains how it monitors my mother's heart rate and stimulates the muscles to contract if there is too much time between heartbeats. She tells us how to send information from her pacemaker to the company over the phone. She shows my mother how to care for the stitches and helps arrange a follow-up visit for any needed adjustments in the pacemaker programming.

After the nurse leaves, my mother and I study the brochure that she has received from the company that manufactured the pacemaker. We carefully review the warnings she has to keep in mind. For example:

- My mother should not hold a cell phone closer than six inches to her new pacemaker.
- My mother should not stand closer than twelve inches to a slot machine.

These are good and reasonable suggestions. Although she rarely uses her cell phone, she does own one. The company suggests that she hold the phone on the ear opposite the device when she needs to make a call. We make a note of that. Since my mother has never been inside of a casino or a tavern, she doesn't need to worry about slot machines. She decides that the company believes that it is safe to play the slots, but big winners must avoid hugging the machine after hitting a jackpot.

We continue reading. My mother laughs out loud when the brochure warns against the following activities:

- My mother should stand no closer than twelve inches to a chainsaw.
- My mother should be no closer than two feet from an arc welder.
- My mother should *never* use either a stun gun or a jackhammer.

These also seem to be very reasonable suggestions, although I tighten my grip on her hand and lock eyes with her. I question her closely, and she repeatedly assures me that she has long ago given up her aspirations to become a lumberjack, welder, peace officer, or road construction worker.

"Can I trust you?" I ask. "Promise that you will let me know immediately if you feel an urge to take up any new hobbies that involve heavy equipment or high-voltage generators." She nods solemnly and we shake on the promise, her skin smooth in my hand, her fingers cool to the touch, her joints swollen, her grip weakened by arthritis.

Despite her insistent claims to the contrary, I continue to monitor her hobbies and activities for the rest of her life. Even after she moves to senior apartments close to our home, I ask her whether she has been to a casino or visited a logging camp.

I surreptitiously check the hallway closet for stun guns and her garage space for jackhammers. She always throws up her hands in mock denial but, with all of that enhanced energy she gained from her new pacemaker, I tell her that I need to be certain.

PART TWO

First Encounters

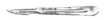

The Code

What we see depends mainly on what we look for.
- John Lubbock

The emergency department staff rarely tracks me down in the middle of the night, so when I see the trauma room callback number on my pager, I flick on the light and dial. *This can't be good.*

"What's up?"

"Mr. Robinson came in a few hours ago, and his family is asking for you. He had been bleeding through his tracheostomy tube off-and-on most of the day. We were getting ready to send him home when he suddenly started coughing out blood again. Do you think you could come in?"

"Yeah, of course." I sit up. "I'll be there in twenty minutes."

I hang up the phone. I am Mr. Robinson's cancer surgeon but have little to offer now other than the knowledge of his treatment; the emergency department staff will be doing all the work. Our visits in the office have become routine, though. He and his family are gentle souls. I anticipate focusing most of my attention on the family.

As I drive to the hospital, I try to recall every detail of his case. Several months ago, I had evaluated him for a large, obstructing laryngeal cancer and performed a tracheotomy. Mr. Robinson, his family, and I had gotten to know each other as we worked through his treatment options.

Now, two months after finally completing a rigorous combination of radiation therapy and chemotherapy, this bleeding heralds a sudden and worrisome turn. Has a blood vessel in the larynx eroded? Is he bleeding from the lower esophagus? Both are serious, yet potentially treatable, problems.

A third scenario places the bleeding source in the upper chest where the tip of his tracheostomy tube might have eroded into one of the large vessels overlying the trachea. A hole that develops directly from a vessel into the airway almost always leads to massive, uncontrollable bleeding. I try to focus on the less lethal possibilities but cannot.

I park and walk directly to the trauma room. As the door slides open, I realize a full code is underway. Bright red blood flies into the air every time the respiratory therapist squeezes on the ventilating bag to force air into his lungs. A stream of blood runs from the tracheostomy site onto the cart below his neck and shoulders. Blood fills suction canisters as the staff tries to keep his airway clear. I ease my way through the crowd, listening as the emergency physician works though the resuscitation protocol. The monitors beep incessantly.

I barely recognize the lanky, unresponsive man on the cart. His half-closed eyes are unfocused and expressionless. His limbs recoil after each chest compression. Despite the blood running through large intravenous lines, there is clearly no way that the transfusions can pour fluids into his body rapidly enough. The room smells strongly of caked and clotting blood.

I look around. Blood is splattered on the equipment, the linens, and the floor. Once in a while, someone wipes Mr. Robinson's face.

The room hums as everyone tackles their assigned roles. A pharmacist draws up medications. Aides run samples of blood to the lab. A radiology tech waits to see if any X-rays are needed. A housekeeper empties bags of bloodied garbage and towels, moving methodically from one container to the next.

"Right after we called you, he suddenly cut loose! We haven't been able to get a pressure for a while." The emergency physician looks at me. "I think it is time to talk to the family. How well do you know them?"

"Pretty well," I acknowledge, glancing up at him and wondering how we will break this to them. "They are good folks."

"Okay," he says. "Let's go have a talk."

I tell the emergency physician what I can remember about the family as we walk down the hall to the family waiting room. Mrs. Robinson grabs my hands when we enter, and I focus on her. "He's alive, but just barely. The doctors and nurses are doing all they can, but he is not responding to the treatments." I look around the room. "I can tell you that he is in no pain. I wish I had better news but, at this point, the bleeding is continuing, and his heart just can't keep up."

A relative begins to sob. "Oh, Lord!" exclaims one of the adult daughters. "He had been getting better! Yesterday was a wonderful day! He was laughing and joking . . . he ate a fish for dinner just before we came in!"

I do not tell them everything. I do not tell them that this tall, imposing man now looks disturbingly pale as he lies on a cart down the hall. I do not tell them about the grim faces of the staff.

And I do not tell them about the blood.

The emergency physician addresses Mrs. Robinson. "Would you like to come into the trauma room and be with him while we work?"

What? My eyes widen, and I turn to look incredulously at the doctor. Although there are protocols in place that encourage families to be nearby during resuscitations, I have never been involved in a code where the family was in the room. Codes can be brutal, sterile, and impersonal affairs, and this code seems unusually surreal because of the blood that coats everything. I worry about the family's reaction.

"Oh, we can go be with him?"

"Absolutely," says the emergency physician. "I am going back in, and Dr. Campbell will bring you in after he tells you what to expect." *How am I to do that, exactly?* I stare behind him as he disappears down the corridor.

I prepare them the best I can. "He's on the cart, and the team is pressing on his chest and helping him breathe," I tell them. "There will be space for you near his feet so you can be near him. I will be there the whole time and will tell you what is going on. If you want to leave, let me know."

A few minutes later, I escort three family members to his bedside, guiding them into positions where they can see yet would still have a ready escape route. I keep my hand on Mrs. Robinson's shoulder and find her a chair where she can hold one of his hands. His sister, comforted similarly by one of his daughters, sits across from us and latches onto an ankle. I watch the family members closely. I narrate the action as the resuscitation attempt continues. He has no pressure, no pulse. Nothing.

My apprehension that the family might become unglued proves completely unfounded. They focus on the patient. I, on the other hand, find myself listening to the team and watching the blood cascade steadily onto the floor.

Several minutes pass. The emergency physician nods at me and then addresses Mrs. Robinson. She listens but did not look up.

"We are going to stop now, okay? This is not helping him. Let's let him rest."

Mrs. Robinson stares intently at her husband's hand as she rubs his fingers steadily between her own. She nods. The chest compressions stop. The staff recedes, and the room goes still.

"Oh, God!" the sister cries out. "Is he dead now?"

The staff rotates the monitors out of view, eventually turning them off. The housekeeper empties a bag of trash. I feel Mrs. Robinson's shoulder heave under my hand as she speaks. "He is at peace now." She continues massaging his fingers.

For several minutes, the family keeps hold of him. The sister's breathing steadies as she rests her head on his legs.

Mrs. Robinson looks up and considers the scene around her. "I'm ready." We file back to the waiting room where, over the next half-hour, their pastor and several family members comfort one another. The news spreads quickly to the extended family.

The rest of the family eventually asks to see him. When we return to the trauma room, the floor sparkles and the room smells intensely of bleach. The housekeeper has done an extraordinary job.

Mr. Robinson, still eerily pale, looks comfortable, head tilted slightly to the left, his eyes closed. His relaxed, supple hands rest outside of the clean sheet covering him. The conversation tentatively returns to mundane things. Mr. Robinson's brother had caught the fish that he had eaten for dinner. "Did he enjoy it?" the brother wants to know. He sure did! The brother beams, and everyone laughs. I look around; there isn't a drop of blood visible anywhere.

The family returns to the waiting room. I thank the emergency department staff and track down the housekeeper. "Thank you. Nice work," I tell her. She smiles and turns away.

Because it is 6:45 a.m., I decide to make rounds before heading to my car. When I finally pull out of the parking structure, the housekeeper is waiting at the bus stop, wearing a warm coat over her scrubs, clutching her bag, and waiting patiently for the ride that will carry her home.

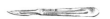

Learning to Fly

Difficulties are things that show a person what they are.

- Epictetus

Within weeks of launching his or her medical career, every newly minted surgeon walks into a room and confronts the biggest tumor, the most complex constellation of findings, or the worst injury he or she has ever faced. The physician's skills are stretched to their absolute limits. Someone's life might be on the line. Someone's career might be in the balance. Journal articles and textbook chapters offer only so much help, and then the case takes another unexpected twist.

One day, shortly after completing my fellowship and entering practice, I encounter a very challenging patient. Although it is difficult to discern by looking at him, our ages are not all that far apart. His face is swollen, his neck and lip bear surgical scars, and his skin is discolored from radiation therapy. A destructive, angry-looking throat cancer has overwhelmed all prior attempts at treatment. His eyes confirm that the growing tumor is his constant tormenter.

Reflexively, I fall back on the same checklists that recently enabled me to survive my board certification exams. First, I review the details of his history and carefully document the physical findings. After studying the laboratory reports, I review his scans. I point to the radiologist's arrows that outline the extent of his cancer. As I study the images, I silently search for clues of whether his disease might yield to yet another surgical procedure.

Both the patient and I have difficult decisions to make. An operation offers him only the slimmest possibility of again becoming cancer-free. Even if successful, the side effects might be overwhelming. From my perspective, any procedure will be incredibly challenging. Although my training has included years of standing across the operating table from a series of very talented surgeons, this case will push the limits of both my experience and my skills. And I will be the one making the decisions.

The patient and his family ask difficult questions. He signs the consent form. It's a go.

As I prepare for the operation, I earnestly wish I could somehow gain access to all of the tricks my mentors discovered throughout their careers. During training, I noticed how instinctively, almost casually, they approached destructive cancers and wickedly distorted anatomy. This case will test, for the first time, how closely I paid attention.

A few days later, we are in the operating room. Within minutes of making the incision, it is clear that my patient's prior treatments have left the tissues rock-hard and impenetrable. Each spread of a hemostat causes more bleeding. Anatomic landmarks are missing, so muscles and nerves appear in unexpected places. Each new challenge brings things to a standstill. *What was I thinking to schedule this?*

Fortunately for me, I have arranged for a trusted senior surgeon to be available to help, if needed. After a couple of hours, he calls into the operating room. "Do you want me to come and take a look?"

"Absolutely!" I answer. "That would be great."

I struggle to recall and apply every lesson and trick I ever learned. *Find anatomic structures and follow them*, I remind myself. *Don't cut anything until you are certain you won't need it later. Don't work yourself into a hole.* I adjust my approach, but progress is still glacial.

My colleague calls again. The OR nurse holds the phone to my ear. "Sorry," he says. "I got tied up. I'll be there in a while."

"That's fine," I say. "Come whenever you can."

I push on. *Maximize exposure*, I remind myself. *Make sure the assistant knows what I am trying to do. Take whatever time the case requires. Think several steps ahead.* I change the angle of attack and come at the cancer again. Still no visit from my senior colleague.

Gradually, though, I make progress. Things perceptibly fall into place and, miraculously, the dissection begins to reveal some recognizable anatomy. The pace quickens. A few well-placed knife strokes and, finally, the surgical field yields the cancer.

The telephone rings again. "Sorry. I'll be there shortly."

"Don't bother. We're closing. Thanks, anyway."

Annie Dillard once noted that, "You've got to jump off cliffs all the time and build your wings on the way down." For several hours, I have watched the rock face rush past me. I have sensed the rustle of air racing through feathers.

My senior colleague smiles and says little the next day.

I will never know if he intentionally left me to struggle. I do know, however, that I can still summon up that mixture of relief and gratitude I experienced the very first time my mentors' voices helped me gain control, level out, and slowly learn to trust the wind.

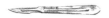

Commencement

Once you really commence to see things,
then you really commence to feel things.
- Edward Steichen

Medical school and residency comprise a long series of "firsts." Consider the neophyte trainee standing at the bedside of a dying woman for the very first time. The young student – who may have never experienced a significant loss in their own life – sits and listens as the woman's husband patiently and unflinchingly shares his grief, revealing the intimate details how his wife's death will impact the family.

Similarly, consider the significance the first time a student steps alone into a clinic room and another human being allows – *expects* – the student to wash their hands and approach the exam table. The student moves aside the patient's gown and listens to the heart and lungs, searches for the liver and spleen, and hunts for signs of illness. Does every student wonder how they will respond if the patient looks into their startled eyes and asks, "What do you think it is? Will I be all right?"

For better or worse, the linear structure of a life in medicine forces students to have many first experiences accompanied by mentors-of-the-moment who are often merely one or two steps ahead of them in training. There is a first time each student or young physician repairs a cut, gives a shot, starts an IV, takes the knife in hand, delivers bad news, hears a murmur, or slides in a catheter. There is a first time they sense the pulsation of an aortic aneurysm, realize that a patient is trying to deceive them, or feel their hand enveloped by the warmth of the abdominal contents. There is a first time when they come up with a correct diagnosis and a first time when they do not. There is a first time another person dies while they wait and watch. Then, there is the first time they observe all of the other students and physicians in the room and figure out how they are supposed to react.

As young adults begin medical school, their "vicarious empathy" – the ability to sense another's feelings, thoughts, suffering, or attitudes – is identical to their peers outside of medicine. Their vicarious empathy drops throughout medical school, particularly after the first and third years, likely because they are being swept along in a maelstrom of difficult experiences with little or no acknowledgement that these are truly momentous, life-altering events. Maybe they stop to ponder. Maybe they shrug. Maybe they have one of these experiences and then move on to whatever subsequent urgent task next awaits them.

Occasionally, someone recognizes that the student or young physician has had a seminal moment and tries to pull him or her off the treadmill long enough to ask, "What just happened here? What are you thinking? Let's talk for a minute." That potential moment of mentorship, sadly, is the exception rather than the rule.

As a result, many students become physicians without the benefit of ceremonies or signposts to mark the accumulating moments that separate them from their future patients. They continue their nearly imperceptible transformations.

Each spring, medical schools hold commencement ceremonies to celebrate their graduates' successful completion of the curricula and to award degrees. Like other institutions of higher learning, there are processions, bunting, speeches, farewells, music, and caps-and-gowns. There is great happiness and celebration as the graduates stand at the cusp of their careers.

I would argue, however, that medical school graduates "commence" long before they receive a diploma. From the day each of them first slips on the white coat until that day, years later, when he or she takes it off for the final time, they experience a perpetual succession of commencements devoid of ceremonial ritual or formal recognition. Without someone to help them recognize the moment, however, the student or young physician learns very early on to walk out of the room after the husband has told them about how his wife's death will devastate their children, take a breath, and get back to work.

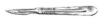

Mistakes

To regret deeply is to live afresh.
- Henry David Thoreau

As a surgeon, I have made mistakes that have hurt people. This should not surprise anyone since, besides being a surgeon, I am also a human being. I have never intentionally hurt anyone in the operating room, but no doctor, nurse, or health care professional is perfect, and our blunders, intended or not, have real consequences. Frighteningly, the National Academy of Medicine estimates that medical errors are the third leading cause of death in the US, trailing only cancer and heart disease.

It gets personal.

Many years ago, I made a horrible mistake and caused permanent harm to one of my patients. The individual had finished cancer treatment and had undergone a follow-up biopsy to determine whether the cancer was, indeed, gone. Another physician went to the lab to check the result and was led to believe that the biopsy had shown that there was persistent cancer.

I was surprised that the cancer was still present but, in a lapse I have regretted ever since, I failed to personally call the pathologist to confirm the unexpected diagnosis. We scheduled the procedure and performed a major operation that changed that individual's life forever. Later, when I learned the truth and realized that I should *not* have performed the operation, I was horrified. Although I was never able to reconstruct exactly what happened, I suspect my colleague had mistakenly located and reported the biopsy report from *before*, rather than *after*, treatment.

Before long, there were lawyers involved. While things were being settled, I apologized repeatedly, tried to be honest and completely transparent. I made an effort to accompany the patient and family. As miserable as I felt, I knew it was immeasurably worse for them.

The experience left me empty at the time and still haunts me decades later. A file containing notes and the legal decision sits in my office and, over the years, I have occasionally pulled it out, reviewed the documents, and checked to see how much they evoke the old churning in my belly and sense of failure. For years, I never talked about the case with anyone.

I recall that particular event with shame. Up to that point, I had always believed that if I studied hard, stayed up to date, listened carefully, communicated openly, cared deeply, documented thoroughly, practiced empathetically, and remained scrupulously ethical, everything would always turn out fine. "Bad things" might happen to *other* doctors, but only because they would never be as compulsive and careful as I intended to be. My patients and I would be invulnerable. It was devastating to learn otherwise, and it haunted me for a long time.

Eventually, and despite my misgivings, I began to share my story with students and trainees, hoping that something good could come from my experience. I reminded them that, as surgeons, our mistakes can have immediate, life-changing consequences. More than simply warning my residents to compulsively double-check unanticipated test results, I hoped they would understand that we are all one small, unintended slip away from disaster, and that the harmful effects fall squarely on the patient and family.

The process of opening up to my residents was, in its own way, cathartic. Despite continuing to regret the harm I caused, sharing my story led me down a path of self-compassion.

I continue to be human. I still make mistakes. I am not afraid to tell a patient that I am sorry. The good news, though, is that I don't believe I have again taken someone else's word on a critical report when the findings did not make sense and the patient's future quality of life hung in the balance.

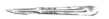

The Sentinel

Experience is a private, very largely speechless affair.
- James A. Baldwin

"Tell me how I will die."

His anaplastic thyroid cancer is "growing audibly," as we sometimes say. This is the worst kind of thyroid cancer, and it is already too large and too widespread for an operation. These tumors often invade the trachea and nearby structures, and almost always kill their hosts in a matter of days or weeks. The CT scan shows innumerable lung metastases. His voice is breathy. He is sitting up in the hospital bed, and any exertion disturbs his breathing. There is an ominously familiar odor in the air.

Over the past few hours, he has just now begun to grasp that his is no ordinary cancer. His voice and face betray his anxiety.

"I mean, what will kill me? What will happen?"

Because of my own anxiety, I retreat to familiar ground to answer. Most of my patients who have no realistic treatment options are dying from less virulent cancers; the conversation with them centers on maintaining the airway, reversing nutritional depletion, and providing support as the disease progresses. Anaplastic thyroid cancer shares these attributes, but it is dramatically more aggressive. These are turbocharged cancers. Disturbing and unwelcome memories well up in me as we talk; I feel a knot in my gut as I recall previous encounters with these unresponsive, destructive, and rapidly fatal tumors. Indeed, several of my patients never left the hospital once the diagnosis was confirmed.

So, I slip into my standard speech that describes what we can do to help any cancer patient. At the same time, my mind scans forward, anticipating what would be an unusually challenging surgical procedure.

"Well, first of all, I suggest that we perform a tracheotomy as soon as we can to make certain that you are able to breathe safely even if the cancer continues to grow. Since you are starting to have more trouble swallowing, I will also help arrange for a feeding tube so you will never have to worry about being able to get enough nutrition and medications."

My gaze shifts back and forth between his eyes and his distorted neck. I am amazed to see how much the mass has enlarged since he had a CT scan two days ago; it reminds me of the overflowing pouch a child might use to contain an ever-growing collection of marbles. I run through mental checklists. One vocal cord has already been paralyzed by the cancer. If the tumor knocks out the other vocal cord, his distress will intensify. The anesthesiologist will struggle to place an endotracheal tube. We will have to excavate through several centimeters of tumor just to find his trachea. The scan confirms that there are large vessels within the mass . . .

"So, if you take care of the breathing and the nutrition, how do the metastases kill you?"

His question snaps me back to the present. A close relative

of his died earlier in the week of extensive cancer. He is frustrated and guilt-ridden that the rest of the family is occupied making arrangements for the funeral while still following his own evolving journey. My patient will have to miss the memorial service while recovering from the planned procedures. The entire family is reeling.

"Well, many of my patients with metastases just get more and more tired. They eventually spend lots of time in bed and often just fall asleep. Our whole team works with you and your family."

Abruptly, he relaxes and, although still sitting nearly upright, closes his eyes.

As he does so, I grit my teeth, knowing that I have omitted sharing another distinct possibility. Anaplastic thyroid cancer often invades and destroys major blood vessels. When the common carotid artery – the major source of blood to the brain – suddenly ruptures, everything in the vicinity – the patient, the room, the bed, the mirror, the furniture, and the caregivers – becomes covered with blood as though sprayed from a renegade fire hose. Few survive.

Even more ominous, a "sentinel bleed" often heralds the impending rupture minutes, hours, or days before the catastrophic event itself. Do I tell him this? Will the angel of death send ripples of terror through him every time he notices a drop of blood in his mouth or on a tissue?

He rests quietly.

We will arrange for the members of the hospice team to see him. They will guide the patient and family through the unknowable and unpredictable days to come. They will offer comfort, support, and care. I will work with them.

I believe that I should warn him of the bleeding event that his body is almost certainly planning. I explore the dusty, dark corners where the memories of past encounters reside. I wonder what the best of my mentors would have shared.

I inhale and run my hands across the rough plastic arms of my chair. He is quiet and peaceful, eyes nearly shut, his head bobbing slightly. I shake my head, exhale, and curse myself for not knowing exactly what to say.

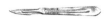

The Phone Call

*Ay, grief goes, fades; we know that – but ask the
tear ducts if they have forgotten how to weep.*
- William Faulkner

Two years have passed since his wife died, and his grief, still
fresh and constantly renewed, continues to consume him. After
trying to make sense of things, he finally writes me a long letter,
three pages of neat, handwritten script, that centers around two
questions. "Why did she die?" he wants to know. "Did someone
do something wrong?" I set the letter down and log into my
computer.

I open her medical record and read through her chart,
recalling her story. She was almost eighty years old when we
met. I remember the couple as having a quiet, old-world charm.
Always neatly dressed, polite, and carrying accents that reflected
their Eastern European upbringing, neither had any of the
habits that are associated with tongue cancer. Neither had ever
smoked. Neither drank any alcohol. All I could surmise was that
she had lived long enough that her immune system was unable
to recognize and fight off her cancer. I remember her husband
as a small, anxious balding man with a gray mustache who wore
sweater vests and herringbone-pattern trousers most of the

time. She said little but, as each visit wrapped up, she would rise from the chair, formally shake my hand, and say, "Thank you, Doctor."

Over the course of two years, her tongue cancers became gradually more aggressive; the last one would have required extensive surgery. Unfortunately, she was not at all healthy and was certainly not interested in the potential risks and side effects of a major procedure.

We reviewed her options, and they chose to pursue a course of radiation. Before the treatment was completed, though, she stopped. "I cannot do this, Doctor," she told me. "It's just too hard. I have lived a good life." She decided against any further active treatment.

A few days later, she was admitted to a hospital closer to her daughter's home. I lost contact with her and her family. She apparently died a few weeks later.

I review the letter once again and then call him. He still has many difficult questions. "Why were the treatments stopped?" "What could have been done differently?" "Why did you give up on her?"

I field his questions as best I can. Then I say, "I have fond memories of her. She was so kind. Tell me what you remember about her."

I listen as he shares his life before and after her death. I knew they had a bakery but had not realized that they spent essentially every hour of every day together, either in the business or at home. They were inseparable.

"How long were you married?"

"Fifty-four years," he replies. "We were great friends. I keep running across her things in the house."

"I am so sorry," I say. "Tell me how you are doing."

His response answers my question only obliquely. "My children keep telling me that I need to get over it. They say that two years is enough. It is very hard."

"She was wonderful," I say.

The questions eventually slow and he brightens a bit. "What other questions do you have?" I ask.

He is quiet on the other end of the line. "I can't think of any."

I picture him in his sweater vest and wonder if he still wears the same pants. I give him my office phone number and ask him to call whenever he wants.

"I might. I feel a bit better. Thank you, Doctor."

Poet Barbara Crooker writes that, "Grief is a river you wade in until you get to the other side | But I am here, stuck in the middle, water parting | around my ankles, moving downstream | over the flat rocks . . . I can't cross over. | Then you really will be gone." There is no set limit on how long we will find ourselves in that river.

"It was good to talk," I tell him. We say goodbye. I tap a few keys on my computer to close her medical record. He never calls again.

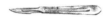

Listening to Leviticus

The fear of death follows from the fear of life.
A man who lives fully is prepared to die at any time.
- Mark Twain

Only, you shall not eat flesh with its life, that is, its blood.
- Genesis 9:4 NRSV

This particular day, more than most, I am working without
a net. Each surgical maneuver intensifies my awareness of the
potential for disaster and uncontrollable bleeding. Repeatedly,
I press forward, making sporadic progress, until I am forced to
back off once again. With each moment of self-doubt, I pause,
regain my focus, and force my hands to return to the procedure,
although my mind begins to doubt whether I should, indeed,
continue.

As I work, the din of the operating room drops away. I twist
my body – leaning hard into the table – and deliberately extend
my right index finger more deeply into the surgical wound.
I focus on the unseen surface of the mass where my finger is
probing and dissecting, hoping for better exposure. Each time I
rearrange my hand or one of the surgical retractors, my eyes scan
the operative field for unexpected surges of blood. I work as

deliberately as possible, proceeding from known to unknown, keeping assistants and supplies ready. If all goes well, with a final sweeping flourish, the softball-sized tumor attached to the inferior end of the right thyroid lobe will soon emerge from the surgical opening like the crowning head of a newborn.

Only then will I know if I exercised good judgment.

I met the man lying on the operating table before me two weeks ago. Physically, he was substantial and rough-hewn, with clear, intelligent eyes and an engaging, peaceful demeanor. Obstructive breathing symptoms had developed slowly over several months, and he gradually noticed more trouble when lying down or holding his head in certain positions. A series of studies revealed a large mass of tissue – a goiter – extending from the bottom of his right thyroid lobe into his upper chest, sharply displacing his trachea. A needle biopsy had found no sign of cancer, but, because of the worsening symptoms, he agreed that the mass would eventually need to be removed. After confirming that the goiter was growing, he had called for an appointment to see me.

During the office visit, we covered the standard discussion of surgical risks. "You know," I said, "there are hazards for all thyroid operations: infection, nerve injury, voice change, problems with the body's calcium levels, lack of improvement, bleeding . . ." I presented each of the potential risks and then discussed prevention and management. "Fortunately, complications are uncommon."

He looked down at his massive hands and then directly into my eyes. "Doctor," he told me, "you have to know that I am a Jehovah's Witness." He smiled and matter-of-factly outlined his convictions without any hint of embarrassment or sign that he was primed for an argument; he readily acknowledged that there might be real and serious consequences if he started bleeding during the operation. I was only too aware that the tenets of his faith prohibit the use of any blood transfusions. Despite the risks, he remained completely serene. On the other hand, my anxiety began to take shape.

The Jehovah's Witnesses' basis for refusing transfusions puzzles those of us outside the faith. Although the use of blood transfusions grew steadily after the 1900 discovery of blood types and compatibility, the prohibition of transfusions was not articulated by the Watchtower Society until 1945. Since then, adherents have stressed both the perceived dangers of transfusions and the benefits of bloodless surgery. To guide the faithful, the church has relied on several biblical texts including Genesis 9:4, Leviticus 17:10-12, Deuteronomy 12:24, and Acts 15:28-29. Although "transfusion" is not mentioned in the Bible, the relevant passages extol the sacredness of blood and warn about the dire consequences of consuming it. For example, God, speaking through Moses in Leviticus, commands the people: "If anyone of the house of Israel or of the aliens who reside among them eats any blood, I will set my face against that person who eats blood, and will cut that person off from the people. For the life of the flesh is in the blood." The biblical texts provide a powerful commandment as well as an ominous warning to the believer.

Before proceeding further, I needed to make certain that my patient and I had a complete understanding. Would he refuse all types of transfusions?

"Yes."

Would he agree to donate blood ahead of time in case we needed to transfuse it back into him at the time of his surgery?

"No, I don't think so."

Could we salvage his own blood, process it, and return it to him during the operation?

"No."

Did he realize that his blood cell count might possibly get so low that it could be very dangerous?

"Doctor, I understand completely that by refusing blood transfusions, I might die. That is the choice I have made, and I am very comfortable with that choice." He paused, and then asked, almost casually, "So, will you do the surgery?"

Now it was my turn to make a choice. The mass was growing; clearly, at some point he would need surgery. His risk for significant blood loss was greater than usual because of the size of his goiter and its extension into the upper chest. His physical size might make access to critical structures difficult. If uncontrolled bleeding began, liters of blood could escape the wound in a very short time. On the positive side, I rarely need to order blood transfusions during thyroidectomies.

But how would I feel if he died a presumably preventable death while in my care? Could I really adhere to his instructions in every possible circumstance? I was not certain.

"Do you want to go over things again?" I asked.

"That won't be necessary, Doctor." He smiled and folded his hands. "I understand and accept all of the risks. I will sign any forms that you require. I have faith, above all, that things will go just as they are meant to go."

I reassessed the scans and ultrasound images while he waited patiently. I exhaled. "Okay," I said, "let's take a look at the schedule."

"The sooner the better, Doctor. I'm ready whenever you are."

Now, two weeks later, this powerful man with the thick neck lies asleep on the operating table. Things are not going as smoothly as I hoped. The muscles have been difficult to separate cleanly from the superficial surface of the thyroid gland, and as I work my way down the neck and into the upper chest behind the sternum, the passageway tightens dramatically. The limited space between the bone of the spine and the bone of the sternum is completely filled by the mass, barely permitting the insertion of a finger. I probe the depths cautiously. I have performed this maneuver enough to realize that, with sufficient effort, the mass should suddenly become free of the surrounding attachments and miraculously appear in the wound, yet I am hesitant to exert more force. *I can't afford to tear a blood vessel,* I think to myself.

As I repeatedly advance my finger into the unyielding space, a firm pressure pushes back at me. I continue to second-guess myself. *Why did I so quickly agree to operate on him?* Had a voice whispered, "Sure, you can do that! No problem!"? I continue dissecting the enveloping tissues from the surface of the gland, working side to side, top to bottom, and front to back, resolutely forcing the tissues apart. From deep within, I hear the old adage, "All surgery ends eventually," and I question whether this one will end well. I push deeper, adding a second finger and extending them both as far as they can reach. A few fibers separate, there is a hint of movement, but the mass stubbornly stays in place. Again, I push. Then again.

Suddenly, something deep and unseen gives way and the goiter noticeably moves upward into the palm of my right hand. As my fingers cradle the mass, I keep steady pressure on the walls

of the unseen cavity. If the final releasing maneuver has torn a
deep, undetected blood vessel, direct pressure will control the
hemorrhage for the time being. As the mass is delivered up and
out of the chest, I fill the space behind it with surgical sponges.
Simultaneously, I reposition my fingers and coax the goiter out
of the wound. My eyes, however, continue to search the space
from which the gland had just emerged.

"Suction, please. More sponges. Keep pressure right there."

I reach overhead and move the operating room lights to
better illuminate the depths, then gradually release pressure,
carefully removing the surgical sponges one by one. A pool of
dark blood appears in the cavity. I stare cautiously as the fluid
level emerges from, and then – thank God – drops back into
the wound, rising and falling in cadence with the ventilator.
For several seconds, I focus on the reflection of the lights on
the meniscus of blood, finally convincing myself that nothing
is welling up from below. Only then does the pounding in my
temples recede, and I can hear the sounds of the monitors and
voices of the OR staff again.

"Irrigation, please." I wash out the wound and control
a couple of small bleeding points, preparing for final closure.
Within minutes, the procedure is complete, and the patient is
wheeled to the recovery room. I stand at the foot of his bed and
watch him until he opens his eyes and nods at me.

I head toward the family center. As I walk, I think back to
the clinic visit when he had placidly reassured me that he was
"prepared to die." For my part, I spent two weeks becoming
increasingly anxious that I might suddenly be called upon to
"protect" this man from his own convictions. What emergent
course of action might I have taken if he had lost a quart of

blood? A gallon? What would it have felt like to carry out his instructions? Would I have eventually tried to convince his family to authorize a lifesaving transfusion? Even after thinking through every possibility in the days leading up to the surgery, I was not certain. Fortunately, things had not come to that.

All I know for certain is that he is going to be fine and that, if the situation ever arises again, I will still be working without a net.

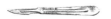

The Transition

Life is pleasant. Death is peaceful.
It's the transition that's troublesome.

-Isaac Asimov

His initial office visit sets the tone for everything that follows; despite all that has gone before and all that is yet to come, he appears serene, almost bemused. The family presents the envelopes that contain his records and, as we review all the paperwork and scans, he quietly watches us interact. I wonder about him; he seems too peaceful, given the dire situation.

Several months ago, he pushed his doctor to biopsy a sore spot on his tongue. His physician was surprised to find that the sore was malignant. He had no risk factors for oral cavity cancer – he never smoked and rarely drank. He was extremely careful about his diet and exercised faithfully.

His initial treatment was a combination of radiation therapy and chemotherapy. A few weeks later, his cancer rapidly reappeared. He comes to me to learn if a surgical procedure will help.

Although the discussion revolves around the plans for cancer treatment, I also explore his personal story. He recently retired and has a wide circle of friends. His family is extraordinarily close. He exercises relentlessly and spends hours on a treadmill or stair machine. He has many outside interests and looks forward to a future when he can explore each of them. The cancer has robbed him of his ability to articulate and, as he struggles to speak, his family instinctively fills in the blanks for him. At each interruption, he nods gratefully. It is a comfortable dynamic.

A rush of testing, scheduling, and planning takes over, and he is soon heading to the operating room. Given the extent of the cancer and its behavior, the salvage effort is a long shot; still, we all hope for the best. During a ten-hour surgery, much of his tongue and part of his lower jaw is removed and then replaced with skin, muscle, and bone from other parts of his body.

The next few weeks are great. He recovers more quickly than expected because of his underlying excellent conditioning, and the news from the pathology laboratory is very encouraging. The light returns to his eyes. He makes steady progress and, before long, is jotting questions on his notepad looking beyond the cancer treatment: When can I travel? Will I be able to drive? When can I eat? When can I start my exercise routine again? What can I expect?

The improvement is short-lived, however. A few months later, he shows signs of deterioration and then, suddenly, has trouble breathing. He is admitted to the hospital, and a scan finds a brand-new cancer invading his windpipe. There are new metastases spreading to the lungs and bones. In the days before the development of targeted immunotherapy agents, meaningful treatment is not possible.

He desperately wants to go home, but his condition worsens. As he drifts in and out of consciousness, he is placed on a ventilator in the intensive care unit.

His family and friends never leave his side. His pastor visits. Old friends come to see him and console his family.

It is soon time to let him go. As has been his long-stated desire, the family agrees to discontinue life support. It is an appropriate, difficult decision made with tears and prayers.

He is sedated, and the breathing machine disconnected. As sometimes happens, though, he continues to breathe on his own, although with effort. He is moved from the ICU to a private room where the family sits in silence around his bed. His death can come at any time.

A funny thing happens, though; he isn't ready to die quite yet. Despite discontinuing both the fluids and the ventilator, he keeps going. Astoundingly, two days stretch to two more days. He is unconscious – serene and quiet – in his bed, breathing slowly, responding to nothing. As his body disposes of the extra fluid he received from all of the IVs while in the ICU, his swelling decreases. If anything, he looks better than he has for weeks.

Family and friends are unsure how to react to this unforeseen, extended time of waiting. Inevitably, the mood shifts and, as the days pass, the tears run dry. The atmosphere around his hospital bed turns first from deep sorrow to a palpable exhaustion and then to a profound sense of peace.

Tentatively at first, the room gradually fills with favorite music, stories, smiles, snacks, and children's drawings. The space transforms imperceptibly from a dwelling where death was staring down from the walls to a sanctuary where everyone is encouraged to joyfully celebrate the guest of honor's soon-to-be-completed journey. His wife recalls that he would sneak off to the basement to watch his collection of old movies. His children chide him for collecting boxes of baseball cards for his daughter, only to keep them from her grasp as their value increased. They reflect on his love of history, his dynamic family life, his long-lasting and deep friendships, and his place within his community. I stop by the room each afternoon and am welcomed into the circle. In their midst, he remains peaceful and imperturbable, breathing quietly as the celebration continues.

One afternoon, five days after he is removed from the ventilator, I stop in for a short visit. Everyone is tired, and the conversation lags. That evening, he stops breathing and quietly dies. One of my residents calls me with the news. It is finally over.

Because of the extended vigil, I know him much better now than I did a week before. I have new insights into his life, passions, and friendships. I am grateful to have been part of the circle sitting at the bedside and hearing the stories.

One of the great privileges of a physician's calling is – often without being truly earned – the opportunity to be present for and surrounded by stories in times of crisis. Thanks to the family's generosity, I now have a bit more insight into the glorious serenity about which I marveled on the day my implacable patient and I first met.

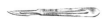

Numb

The capacity to give one's attention to a sufferer is a very rare and difficult thing; it is almost a miracle; it is a miracle.
- Simone Weil

I walk down the steps of the funeral home, squinting as I reach the bright afternoon sun. People move all around me, pushing strollers, walking dogs, searching pockets for car keys, talking on phones, looking into store windows, laughing. They are oblivious.

My mother and I have spent the past hour at the mortuary, making arrangements for my father's remains. The funeral director worked steadily though his list: What should be in the obituary? Should the paper run the listing for two days or three? Here are several forms we need to complete. Could you please sign here? And here? Would you like to pick up the ashes or should we deliver them to the church? Do you want the clothes he was wearing? Because he was a veteran, he is eligible for a flag. We are so sorry for your loss. Will you be paying with a check or credit card?

As I leave the funeral home, I wonder how all of these people could be going about their business as though nothing has happened. Doesn't everyone feel this numbness – this incredible weight – just as I do? How can they be rushing about at such a time?

Each of us is periodically overwhelmed by personal or shared loss. Like most people, I will slowly return to "normal," shaking loose the shroud that is currently pressing down upon me. For years, though, the sensation will revisit me at the most unexpected moments, washing over me like an ocean wave – reappearing in response to a song, a scent, or a fleeting glimpse of something disappearing around the corner – and stopping me dead in my tracks for just a moment.

Cataclysmic experiences like my experience at the funeral home transpire every day in every hospital. It is possible that the man in this room has been given terrible news. A woman in that room might suddenly have realized that her husband is never coming home. Just down the hall, a young family could be coming to terms with a series of difficult and life-altering treatments. Next to the nursing station, a young child is being led to a bedside, perhaps to say goodbye.

One of my patients was admitted overnight after being seen in the emergency room, and I stop in to see him. After finally agreeing several weeks ago that his cancer would best be controlled if I removed his voice box, he struggled both physically and emotionally. His surgery was complicated and his recovery difficult. He is in constant pain, which he recognizes is only partly physical. He is refusing to undergo radiation treatments and chemotherapy, even though he knows they offer him the best opportunity to be cancer-free. He lands in the emergency room every few days for one of a variety of issues. Today, he sits propped in his bed as I enter the room, glancing up at me with a drawn and crestfallen face.

"Good morning," I say. "Are you breathing better today?"

He shrugs and nods. Although he has a voice prosthesis, he prefers to gesture or write.

"What do you want to talk about?"

He pulls out a notepad and begins. Each topic is addressed, but the restoration of health and the return to a strong and independent quality of life seem far off and impossible to achieve. His list is a bit different this week than it was last week. It will change, yet again, by the time I see him in the office next week. I watch as he writes, believing that the surgery has placed in his road what must seem to him several insurmountable obstacles, yet knowing that the extent and pace of his cancer offer no realistic treatment alternatives. I do my best to be fully present to him, and yet, as much as I want to help, and as attentive as his family has been, it seems as though he is fighting a lonely, impossible battle.

I slip back out of his room and run into a colleague. We have a trivial conversation. I hear laughter from a group of residents around the corner. I plot out the rest of my day, trying to save enough time to grab lunch between surgical cases. I make a mental note to call the speech pathologist and one of the pulmonologists to address some of my patient's concerns, yet his issues weigh less on me as I head toward the stairwell. My mind turns to other things.

As I walk down the hallway, I imagine that some of the people within these rooms are waiting for scan results, hoping for a good report from the pathology lab, recalling times when their bodies were intact and energetic, listening for hints of optimism in the nurse's voice, waiting for someone to finally explain what is going on, or coming to grips with the worst possible prognosis. This might be the day when they go numb. I watch as a medical student knocks, calls out the name of the patient within, and slips through the doorway to offer a bit of news.

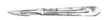

After the Biopsy

It seems to me we can never give up longing and
wishing while we are thoroughly alive.
- George Eliot

She grips my hand. Hard.

"Doctor, what does this mean?"

She is looking for honesty. I have been her physician for ten years and she has fought off cancer twice, first with radiation and then with surgery. Now her cancer has returned.

"Doctor, my grandchildren are just now growing up."

She is looking to the future. She is in her seventies and in good health, but she senses threatening clouds gathering.

"Doctor, I want to go back home to visit my sister."

She is looking at the present. She wants to spend time with her far-distant sibling before it is too late for each of them.

"Doctor, you have helped me before."

She is looking to the past. She hopes that good fortune and technology can sustain her once again.

"Doctor, please."

She looks at me intently. She grips my hand. Hard.

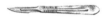

Transience

Hospitals are a little like the beach. The next wave comes in, and the footprints of your pain and suffering, your delivery and recovery, are obliterated; the sheets are changed.
- Anna Quindlen

When a person is hospitalized for more than a few days, the room often takes on his or her personality. For a while, the patient and family have a space – four walls, a bathroom, a window – that becomes their own. I notice the novels, the hometown newspaper, the favorite slippers, the snacks from home, and grandchildren's artwork. When I walk the halls, memories stir as I link specific rooms with particular patients and their stories.

When I was first in practice many years ago, I was asked to see a woman who had spent weeks in the hospital.

She is holding her own but, in the days before hospice, she has nowhere else to go. As I open the door, I am struck by the scent of the flowers within. There is soft music playing on a cassette tape player. The bulletin board is covered with family photos and get-well cards. A handmade "We Miss You!" banner hangs from the ceiling. Board games are stacked on the window ledge.

The place feels like someone's home or maybe their summer cottage. Family and friends have transformed the few square feet of hospital and planted their own personal healing garden.

"The flowers are beautiful!" I comment, approaching the bed rail.

"It's a bit like a funeral parlor, don't you think?" she responds. Her wink and mischievous grin tell me she is only partly serious.

I point to the line of stuffed animals on a shelf. "A very classy funeral parlor," I agree.

Over the coming days, her light dims. Her family keeps vigil, personalizing and rearranging the photos, cards, and mementos.

One day, I knock on the door and peek in. I blink. The fragrance has dissipated, and the room is empty. The bed is raised to its highest setting, and the sheets are crisply made. The room has been reset for the next patient.

She is gone.

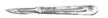

Crystal Ball

*It's strange how the worst day of your life
often starts just like any other.*

- Joanna Cannon

I prepare for each clinic by reviewing the tests and scans of the patients who will be seen that day. Today, I am dismayed as I read a report for a long-standing patient. The news is not good – his scan shows that his cancer has returned. I pause before I enter, preparing what I will tell him.

Twenty years ago, on a day exactly like today, I had the same sinking feeling as I examined a woman with a recurrent cancer. *This is really bad*, I thought to myself at the time. I looked at the CT scans again, staring at the new masses in her neck and in her lungs. *That seals it*, I thought at the time. *This is not curable.*

As I prepared to have that difficult conversation years ago, I ran through my "bad news" checklist: Be fully present. Sit down and lean forward. First ask what she knows. Fire a "warning shot." Be honest yet compassionate. Never smother all hope.

Offer help and support. At the end, review to make certain that everyone understands what was said.

"What do you know about the cancer?" I had asked. "How are you feeling these days?"

"Tired, I guess," she had replied, "but overall, really not too bad. The mass in my neck is getting sore."

I had looked at her and the gathered family. "I have some difficult news we need to discuss."

Talking to patients about a new or recurrent cancer diagnosis is a difficult task. As patients often attest, we sometimes don't do it very well. Over the next few minutes, I reviewed what I had discovered on the scans. We reviewed the images and reports together. "The options are very limited. Surgery will not be helpful, and we cannot give much more radiation therapy. Chemotherapy is possible and might slow the tumor growth but has little chance of curing the cancer."

She had lurched upright in the examination chair. Not defiant, exactly, but intense and animated. "What are you saying, Doctor? Am I dying? I feel fine. Are you saying that I'm terminal? Can't you do something?"

I had looked at her. "The cancer will continue to be with you, but we don't have anything that will cure this. We will do everything possible to support you."

We had covered a lot of territory with questions from both the family and the patient. I let them ask everything that came to mind and promised to get them all of the answers I could. After several minutes, they decided that driving from their home an hour away was a burden and she wanted to see a doctor closer to where she lived to discuss palliative chemotherapy. I called an oncologist I knew. We said goodbye. I never saw her again.

There are always risks when we try to predict how individual patients will do. As anyone who has ever heard a "The doctor told Mom she would be dead in three months and that was ten years ago," story will attest, cancer prognostication is an imperfect science. Large clinical research trials and population-based cancer survival curves tell us what percentage of people with a certain stage of disease will be alive in three or five years. We are never as confident when making predictions for individuals and, back when I had the difficult conversation with my patient, the odds of her long-term survival were essentially zero.

Two years after our difficult conversation, my patient with the incurable cancer sent me a card. She was alive and doing well. Chemotherapy had completely cleared every sign of cancer from her body. She was a cancer outlier.

She chastised me for being so pessimistic about her future and for telling her that she would receive only temporary benefit from any treatment. "You should never tell a patient that they will die," she scolded. "That is a terrible thing to tell someone."

As I wrote her a congratulatory note, it made me wonder – what should I have said? Is it fair to tell everyone in her situation that there is a chance, even if infinitesimal, that everything will turn out just fine? I sometimes say, "I don't know if you will die of the cancer, but I know that when you do die, you will still have the cancer." Of course, I never know anything with one-hundred percent certainty.

We can't explain everything that happens either inside or outside of medicine. "Absolute certainty" isn't part of our repertoire. We work with ambiguity. We teach medical students that medicine is, at times, a world of "awe and mystery." My patient's unexpected cure was one such moment for me.

Since then, cancer response to treatment has become, if anything, even less predictable. Molecular targeting and personalized medicine have become game-changers for certain patients, taking some individuals from near-certain death to complete cures.

I always try to keep in mind that a well-known study comparing two groups of patients with terminal lung cancer found that the group receiving supportive care alone lived longer and reported better quality of life than a group that received palliative chemotherapy. For some patients, it appears that doing nothing is better than doing something.

What is clear is that the correct treatment given to the correct patient whose cancer has the appropriate molecular targets at the correct time in the correct dose might sometimes lead to the complete disappearance of that individual's cancer. But then again, it is also clear that the treatment might be ineffective, colossally expensive, and toxic.

I walk into the exam room where I must share awful news with my patient. My experiences with the patient with the unexpected cancer cure, the development of new treatments, and the availability of clinical trials affect how I approach patients. For this man, though, there are no active clinical trials, and we don't know if he has any immunotherapy options. I recall my patient from twenty years ago and prepare my "bad news" checklist. The conversation today will be different yet the same. He and his family will be devastated and anxious. I will try to be honest and compassionate. If he asks, I will predict the future while preserving hope.

Despite this, I know I can never be certain of anything.

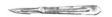

To Enable Well-Being

"When there's no place for the scalpel,
words are the surgeon's only tool."
- Paul Kalanithi, MD

Mrs. Jordan, a withered leaf of a woman, sits crumpled in the clinic exam chair as I introduce myself to everyone. Her husband and daughter are serious, substantial people who shake hands firmly. Mrs. Jordan's grip barely registers.

"The doctors back home have her on chemo," her husband tells me. "We're in a holding pattern." He looks at her. "She wants to keep fighting."

"That's terrific," I respond. "Good for you. So, how can I help?"

I know she is visiting several medical centers after having learned that her cancer has recurred. Her prior surgeon has told her that she is not a candidate for another operation. I am certain they have come hoping my answer will be different.

Having been through surgery, radiation therapy, and chemotherapy for her aggressive tongue cancer, Mrs. Jordan whispers that she has adopted a healthier lifestyle. "I quit smoking! Hardest thing I ever did. We stopped going to fast food restaurants, I walk every day and am being positive. My family and prayer partners are right there whenever I need them." She smiles at her husband. "I'm doing everything the doctors tell me to do."

"She's a trooper!" he says.

The daughter grips her pen. There are several questions on her notepad, and she fills in the blank spaces as we talk. They ask about the cancer and its treatment. What might we offer? What are the risks, given that she is so weak? How urgent is it? Her husband leans forward, raising his eyebrows whenever I pause to frame my responses.

"Before I make any recommendations," I tell her, "let me examine you."

I wash my hands and run through my routine. I aim my headlight and feel inside her mouth. She winces and I apologize. "That's okay, Doc. Do what you gotta do."

The cancer is rock-hard and attached firmly to her lower jaw. I prod and press against the mass, determining where I would need to make incisions and what structures would need to be removed. As the extent of the recurrence comes into focus, I mentally outline a larger and more complex operation. The lymph nodes in the upper neck are enlarged, firm, and full of cancer. Her tongue is partially replaced with the cancer. I look at her voice box and can see that the cancer is creeping down the wall on the inside of her throat. Each tentacle compounds the complexity of a procedure, although I can still envision a potential way to remove everything and offer a reconstruction. Based on what I can see and feel in her mouth and neck, surgery still offers a slim chance for a cure, although she would need additional treatment beyond an operation.

"The physicians at the other hospital ordered some new scans a couple of days ago," the husband says. "Have you seen them?"

"No. Not yet. Let's pull them up and see what they tell us."

I log into the computer and retrieve the images. I scroll through the neck scan and point out where the tongue and jaw are destroyed. I point out the large lymph nodes in the neck. I don't see anything in the neck that I wouldn't have predicted from the examination. The cancer is extensive, but surgery remains an option.

The CT scan of the chest is in a different file. I open it and scroll from top to bottom. I look back and forth between the scan and the report. *Uh, oh.*

I point out what the radiologist discovered. "So," I begin, "this is the scan of your chest." I orient them to the structures on the screen. "These are your lungs. Most of the lung tissue is fine but – look here and here – there are several new masses the radiologist says are growing when compared to the last scan a few months ago." I look at her to see if she understands. "Even though we don't yet have a biopsy, I'm afraid that the cancer has spread to the lungs. These are metastases." I pause and see her sink back into the chair. "I wish I had different news for you, but when these cancers spread to the lungs and other parts of the body, a big surgery is almost never the best option. We need to look into other types of treatment."

The daughter puts down her pen. "What do you mean?" she asks. "No surgery?"

"Even with an operation, the cancer would continue to grow in these new places. We need to address the entire body, not just the mouth."

The patient and her family are silent. The news they likely feared most has arrived.

For many years, my approach at this point in the conversation was to quote statistics and send the patient off to the medical oncologist with an optimistic but noncommittal, "We won't know if chemotherapy works until we try," leaving the most difficult part of the conversation to others.

Palliative care physician Susan Block, MD, quoted by surgeon-writer, Atul Gawande, MD, in his book, *Being Mortal*, chides physicians who dwell on statistics and arrange for endless courses of treatment. "We focus on the facts and the options. But that's a mistake," Block writes. Individuals face different struggles, but the biggest issues are dealing with death, avoiding suffering, protecting loved ones from worry, and avoiding financial ruin. "You're not determining whether they want Treatment X or Treatment Y . . . you're trying to learn what's most important to them."

As I sit in the exam room with Mrs. Jordan and her family, I am acutely aware that we met only a little while ago and she is not really my patient. Yet, the words I have shared have opened a gaping chasm at their feet. I tentatively ask, "What do you understand about your situation, and how do you think you might want to spend your time if your health worsens?"

She is quiet, but then looks up. "Well, I knew when we came in here that the cancer was getting worse," she says. "My hope and dream?" She points to her neck. "I want to be cured of this!" Then, she smiles at her family. "But, if that's not going to happen, my goal is to spend as much time as possible with the grandchildren. And I would love to see my cousins in Florida." Her daughter nods. The family shares some stories about the kids. The husband chuckles. It feels like a start.

We talk until all of the blanks on the notepad have been filled and the daughter's pen is tucked away. Mrs. Jordan says she wants to learn more about her chemotherapy options, so they stop at the desk on the way out to set up a medical oncology appointment.

Gawande writes, "We've been wrong about what our job is in medicine. We think that our job is to ensure health and survival. But really it is larger than that. It is to enable well-being." I like that. Attending to well-being rather than survival requires me to listen and find out what makes life worthwhile for my patients. The discussions are not easy, but with some practice, I hope I am getting better.

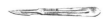

Chocolate and Liquor

Silent gratitude isn't much use to anyone.
- GB Stern

His life revolves around his family, his traditions, and his wheelchair. As a young man in Russia, he lost one leg to war. As an older man, he lost the other to severe blood vessel disease. Now, as an immigrant who speaks no English, he is dependent on his daughter to push him from place to place as she explains all of the inscrutable American customs he encounters along the way. I think he finds us all to be very amusing.

Like many other Russians of his generation, he has loved his vodka, his cigarettes, and traditional foods including *bublitchki*, pickled herring, and borscht. According to his daughter, he had always been robust and energetic despite his disabilities but, in the months before I met him, he lost his spark, and his voice changed from a joyous baritone to a coarse whisper. The growing cancer took away his voice and affected his swallowing. His eyes betray a fear that the things he loves deeply might soon be taken from him.

Treatment is rough. A four-hour surgery keeps him in the hospital for several days. After recovering at home, he endures six challenging weeks of radiation therapy. In the months that follow, he looks deflated and can neither talk nor eat. He needs a feeding tube and becomes completely dependent on his family. He appears intensely discouraged.

Gradually, though, things turn around, and over the next few months, he brightens. His voice returns – maybe not to the rich tones his daughter remembers from her own youth, but to the point where he can sing the old folk songs to his grandchildren. His swallowing and sense of taste improve. He is able to eat many of the foods he remembers from his homeland. Some of the touch points of his world have, at least in part, returned. As he recovers, he becomes more and more enthusiastic.

One day, his daughter wheels him into the clinic for a routine exam. He sits with his coat across his lap as I look in his throat and examine his neck. "You are doing very well," I say. "The cancer is completely controlled. Everything is fine." I give him an exaggerated smile to try to convey my own happiness.

He waits to get the news from his daughter, his eyes moving anxiously from my face to hers as he hears my words interpreted into his mother tongue.

"*Vsyo budyet khorosho*," she reports in Russian as she claps her hands together. "Good news, Papa!"

He smiles broadly and reaches underneath his coat, pulling out a paper bag he has hidden there. From within, he pulls a gift and presses it into my hands with surprising force.

"*Spasiba!*" he exclaims and slaps my shoulder.

"He is saying, 'Thank you!'" his daughter repeats.

I peer into the bag and pull out a small box of specialty chocolates and the pint of liquor. "I can't accept this," I protest. "Please. This is not necessary." I struggle for words. "I'm merely doing my job!"

The daughter intervenes. "Doctor, please understand, this is my father's tradition. Good news is always celebrated with chocolate and alcohol. You have given us the best news possible today! My father wants to share his celebration with you. Please accept! He truly will not understand if you do not." He nods and smiles.

"Really?" I ask. "This is very kind but completely unnecessary."

I reflect on the situation. Celebrate good news with some European chocolate and a bottle of Goldschläger? *What a concept!* It only takes another moment for things to come into focus. "Hmmm," I decide. "This seems like a remarkably fine tradition!"

I open the box of chocolates and offer them to the others in the room. "*Spasiba*?" I repeat back to him. He laughs.

He does not bring gifts every visit, but often enough, to be sure. Colleagues with whom I share the chocolates frequently wonder whether or not I might ask him to return a bit more frequently for checkups.

I have had several thousand patients pass through my practice over the years, and I remember some much better than others. Some, I do not remember at all. However, one of the most memorable was the wheelchair-bound, Russian-speaking survivor of both war and cancer who celebrated good news with chocolate and a toast.

Spasiba, I think again and, sadly, *dasvidaniya*.

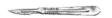

Impact

Seeing, hearing, feeling are miracles.
- Walt Whitman

The nearly blind man is led to a chair in the examination area of the San Salvador clinic where I am working with a small cadre of nurse practitioners, dentists, and other American and Salvadoran physicians. The lines stretch out the door and we are doing our best. This is my first overseas humanitarian trip and, as an otolaryngologist, I quickly discover that few of the people have problems related to their ears, noses, or throats. In fact, it is soon apparent that most of the ailments, whether they are stomach aches, headaches, coughs, or rashes, are as likely to be results of the grinding poverty, the constant menace of violence, and systemic inequity as they are physical issues.

One of our interpreters sits with me long enough to figure out what the man wants. Not only is he nearly blind, we find that he is also quite deaf.

"How can we help you?" the interpreter shouts in Spanish.

The man responds in Spanish. "I have a cough, and sometimes I get headaches," the interpreter repeats. "Can you check me?"

"Sure," I say. "Let me take a look." The interpreter moves

on to work with another member of our team while I perform an examination.

The man is elderly, but it is difficult for me to guess how old he is exactly. His face is deeply lined, and he has a magnificent, gray mustache. He wears an old hat emblazoned with the logo of El Salvador's leftist political party. I can see he has untreated cataracts. I focus my light in his mouth. His few remaining teeth are in terrible shape. Otherwise, his throat looks healthy. The neck is okay. His lungs are clear, and his heart is steady. His belly is soft, and his ankles are not swollen. There are no obvious explanations for either his headaches or his cough but – based on my limited memory of things unrelated to the ears, the nose, and the throat – I don't see anything else seriously wrong, either.

He hasn't complained about his hearing, but that is something I can evaluate even with the limited supplies available. I pull out my otoscope and peek in his ears. Both are completely blocked with wax.

"Would you like me to clean your ears?" The interpreter is tied up elsewhere, so I peek at my cheat sheet with a few Spanish phrases. "*¿Limpia las orejas?*" I venture. I point at his ear.

I'm not at all certain he hears, much less understands, my question. I wonder if I have chosen the correct word for "ears." Nevertheless, he shrugs, turns his head, and offers his ear to me.

Cleaning ears is something I have done regularly throughout my training, although I always used a high-tech microscope, magnification, and suction. This is a decidedly low-tech approach, as he sits in a molded plastic chair next to mine and waits patiently for me to steady my headlight and insert a thin metal curette in his ear canal.

The firm, dark wax is very adherent. As I continue to work the wax away from the edges, he becomes increasingly uncomfortable. He squirms a bit and grimaces. He raises his hand as if to tell me that he had had enough.

Just as I am about to abandon the effort, the plug of wax moves. He appears to sense the change, as well, and his hand settles back into his lap. He again offers his ear. I reset my instrument and slowly work the solid mass of wax from deep within the canal toward the opening.

Suddenly, and triumphantly I might add, I pull out the biggest plug of earwax I have ever seen. It is as big around as a pencil and at least an inch long. Clearly, he has been working on this masterpiece his entire life. Now it is out.

He gasps and then blinks at me with his softened gaze. I ask him, *"¿Tiene dolor, señor?"* Had I hurt him? He frowns. Given the size and density of the wax plug that is now sitting in the gauze on my table, I am certain that his ear canal is very tender. I also suspect that he is hearing from that ear for the first time in many, many years.

"The other?" I attempt in Spanish.

He grins and turns his head to present the other side. Soon, despite more grimacing and hand gestures, I deliver another plug of wax even larger than the first. He focuses his gaze on the wax plugs, shakes his head, and wrings my hand enthusiastically. *"¡Muchas gracias!"* he says.

"*De nada.* You are welcome. Thank you for coming!" Pretty soon, he has received a flu shot and, after waving to me from the doorway, is heading home.

As an otolaryngologist who remembers very little about general medicine, I admit I was out of my depth when patients in El Salvador had concerns about diabetes or heart disease. When those questions arose, I tracked down one of the Salvadorans or Americans so, and as a result, I'm not certain I helped very many of the people during our trip. However, I am very certain there is one nearly blind gentleman who is very, very happy he decided to visit a certain free clinic in San Salvador that day several years ago.

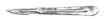

The Sign

*Give, give, give --- what is the point of having experience,
knowledge, or talent if I don't give it away? Of having stories
if I don't tell them to others? . . . It is in giving that I connect
with others, with the world, and with the divine.*
- Isabel Allende

"Dr. Campbell, this is Maurice's sister, Tanya," says the
caller. "I have something I want to bring to your office to give
you."

"Okay," I respond, uncertain what to expect. Maurice was a
long-term patient of mine who died several months earlier after
losing an extended battle with tongue cancer. I have met Tanya
briefly and only once. She gives no clue as to why she wants to
see me. I do not know whether or not to be nervous.

On the appointed day, she stops by my office carrying a
small bag. We talk about Maurice, her only sibling. The family
was close-knit, and she confirms that he had been a loving,
gentle, and hard-working perfectionist.

Maurice spent his working life employed by the county
doing physically and technically demanding jobs. His career
had been cut short when, in the prime of life, he had developed
a tongue cancer. Following surgery and radiation, he did well

for several years. Unfortunately, the cancer returned. Despite more surgery and additional radiation and chemotherapy, the cancer grew over the course of several months. He had reluctantly stopped working and, eventually, there were no more options. He found peace and prepared for the end of his life.

Tanya sits and explains how she and Maurice differed. He was always pragmatic, she tells me, an attitude that did not change even as the cancer progressed. Consistent with his approach to life, Tanya remarks that his approach to death was "rational" and "logical."

I tell her I am not surprised by this. During his office visits, Maurice was always upbeat and analytical, even as we discussed very specific details of his cancer and its treatment. I recall one visit near the end of his life when we had a frank discussion about dying as though we were talking about someone else.

Tanya tells me that she, on the other hand, had struggled mightily as his death approached. Compared to Maurice, she is a devoutly spiritual person who views life and its transitions through a very different lens. "He knew that about me, of course," she says, "so he wasn't surprised when I kept asking him to send a sign when he was safely on the other side."

I am intrigued. *Is this why she has come to see me?* "What did he say to that?" I ask.

"He was a man of few words," she smiles. "Whenever I asked, he nodded but never said much. Late one evening a few days before he died, though, he gave me an answer. 'Remember when you asked for a sign?' he said. 'Of course,' I replied. 'A white butterfly,' he said. He never mentioned it again. I didn't know what to think."

I try to imagine Tanya's reaction. A butterfly? It was the middle of winter in Wisconsin. Had he said something just to appease her? In any case, Maurice died a few days later.

She continues. "So, when I returned from the visitation at the funeral home, a magazine was in the mailbox," she tells me. "I flipped it open, and the first article I saw was illustrated with dozens of white butterflies." From her bag, she pulls a framed copy of the illustration, and we look at it together. "I want you to have this to remember him. This is for you."

I take the gift from her. "Wow," I say. "Thank you very much. I am speechless."

In medicine, we claim to be anchored by certainty and precision but, if we look carefully, we notice moments we cannot explain; all sorts of things that fall outside of our scientific, rational, and logical world. As Anais Nin wrote, "The possession of knowledge does not kill the sense of wonder and mystery. There is always more mystery."

The picture remains on my bookshelf, reminding me of Maurice and Tanya. I still don't know exactly what to think of the white butterflies, but I remain grateful for the gift and for the life it represents.

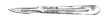

Two Points Along an Arc

The person I miss most is the one I could have been.
- G. B. Shaw

A little boy is running circles around his mother as she stands outside the restaurant smoking a cigarette. I watch them as I walk from the parking lot toward the entrance. The young woman, who appears to be in her twenties, and her friend engage in an animated discussion, the smoke rolling from their mouths and drifting past their faces. Suddenly, the toddler stops running and squeezes his mother's hand. She looks down and, once her gaze has focused on him, he smiles broadly. She grins back at him, tousles his hair, and he resumes running laps. She takes a drag on her cigarette and picks up the conversation where she left off.

A few days later, I am standing at the bedside of a delightful woman in her mid-fifties. Her smoking-related cancer required removal of her voice box and a course of radiation therapy. Months later, her cancer returned with a vengeance. Chemotherapy offered only a temporary reprieve. She is dying.

She is at peace, slipping in and out of wakefulness. The end is near. Her whole family has been preparing for this day, and her adult children gather in a semicircle around the bed. One of her boys sits dejectedly in a chair gripping her hand. Slowly, she awakens, and their eyes meet. He brightens visibly and tightens his grip. She closes her eyes again and they continue to smile, waiting together in silence. It is a powerful moment.

I am struck that the two scenes are essentially from the same drama, with the second following inexorably from the first. Within a few days, I have witnessed two points along the same arc.

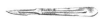

Back in Tune

*[Music] makes practically everyone fonder of life
than he or she would be without it.*
- Kurt Vonnegut

Had I possessed any musical talent whatsoever, my life
probably would have gone in a different direction.

Not that my parents didn't try to turn me into a musician.
They transported me to piano lessons, percussion lessons, and
voice lessons. They bought me a guitar. They pushed me to sign
up for the middle school orchestra and the high school choir.
They encouraged me to join ensembles and audition for the
high school musicals. In retrospect, each exposure enhanced my
appreciation for music but none of the opportunities, by any
stretch of the imagination, created a musician.

My patient, a talented jazz artist, agrees that he knew lots of
kids like me – "eager but musically inept" (his words) – during
his decades-long high school teaching career. Now that he has
retired, he still enjoys performing regularly with a local big
band. Playing his horn is as natural to him as breathing. Music
remains an integral part of his life.

When he develops a throat cancer, I worry that whatever
treatment we propose will close out his playing days. Surgery

will change the shape of the pharyngeal cavity. Radiation will cause severe dryness. I share my concerns with him, and he shakes his head. "Do what you have to do," he tells me. "I'll take my chances."

We decide on a course of treatment. It is not easy. His mouth and throat are forever changed. Each visit shows that the tissues are healing, but it is a slow process.

After a few weeks, he asks, "When can I start playing again?"

"Go ahead and see what happens," I reply. He smiles in a way that betrays the fact that his horn is already getting a workout.

At each follow-up visit, we talk about his progress. "I can play! I need to drink more water, but my chops are returning!"

After a while, he is back performing with the band. Without actively thinking about the process, he has not only recovered from treatment but has compensated for his new physical challenges in ways that I could have never predicted. As I sit in the audience listening to the band one night, I realize that he is playing with confidence. I am relieved.

I try to imagine what it must be like to pick up an instrument and improvise as effortlessly as some of my naturally gifted friends, patients, and colleagues. I am grateful when they share their gifts with the rest of us. And, I guess I am also grateful that my parents finally stopped pushing me to take music lessons and suggested that I consider a different line of work.

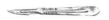

Silent Night

*Sometimes one creates a dynamic impression by saying
something, and sometimes one creates as significant
an impression by remaining silent.*
- Dalai Lama

My patient returns for her annual December follow-up
clinic appointment dressed to the nines and offering hugs and
kisses to everyone in sight. She has been cancer-free for a long
time – many years, in fact – but makes a point to tell me how
much she enjoys these visits, especially the part when I tell
her that everything looks great. I walk into the examination
room and she smiles. Her boots are wet from the snow in the
parking lot.

"How are you doing?" I ask. "You look beautiful, as always!
A vision of loveliness . . . that's what you are!"

She drops her eyes demurely and flutters her fingers at
me, scolding me for flirting and attempting to deflect the
compliment ever so slightly. She is well past eighty and has been
listening to my banter for a long time.

"Have you noticed anything that worries you?" I ask.

She shakes her head. She knows that "nothing new" is good.
She looks great. No new masses. The tongue is soft. The throat

is well healed and open. The neck has no enlarged lymph nodes, and the scars are all stable. The stoma – the opening where her windpipe had been sewn directly to the lower neck skin when her voice box was removed – is open and clean. No changes since the last visit. I jot down a few notes.

"What else is going on in your life?" I ask. "Any trips? Has your family been up for a visit?"

She gestures and tries to coax out some words. As always, I can only pick up a fraction of what she is trying to tell me. "Did you bring your electrolarynx today?" She shrugs and smiles sheepishly. She never brings along her speech device; the batteries are always dead, or she has misplaced it again. She has never liked the buzzing sound. She never wanted a speech restoration procedure.

She digs in her bag for a tiny pencil stub and a dog-eared spiral notebook. She concentrates as she writes out her responses in capital letters. Writing has been her only means of communicating since her voice box was removed at another hospital over twenty years ago. The hospital where the surgery was performed has closed, and her original caregivers have retired. Yet, here she is, silent and unchanged. A cancer survivor.

When I had first met her and skimmed through the faded records, I realized that if she had developed her voice box cancer when I met her instead of two decades before, her treatment would not have included surgery at all. Sometime after her procedure, a clinical research trial demonstrated that treatment with chemotherapy and radiation was just as likely to cure her stage of larynx cancer as an operation. Her physicians, acting on the best information available at the time, though, had removed her voice box, changing her world forever.

She continues to carefully write messages on the lined paper. She writes that her family will come to visit next summer. She writes that her son is doing better. She writes to tell me that she looks forward to these yearly visits. She writes that she is doing okay.

The appointment is over, and she prepares one last message in her notebook in large block letters. "MERRY CHRISTMAS!" it reads. She holds it up and smiles.

"Merry Christmas to you, too," I say. "Have a wonderful year!"

Silent Night is playing over the speaker system as she enthusiastically gives me a hug. Then she slips on her coat and moves down the hall, waving one more time before she disappears around the corner.

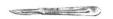

Waiting in Line

At its best, medicine is a service much more than a science.
- Paul Farmer, MD

Long lines form when the global health team arrives. In El Salvador, people arrive in the backs of trucks and then wait hours for one of our provider groups to assess their stomach pains, headaches, or dental problems. The men, all in long pants despite the heat, talk while women in bright dresses tend to the children. In rural Kenya, women in cotton print wraps and men in tattered clothes come from all directions by foot, bicycle, or *"boda boda"* (the ubiquitous motorcycle taxis), waiting on long benches in the equatorial sun. At the medical center in Eldoret, Kenya, the hallway adjacent to the ENT Clinic is packed with people from throughout the region wearing US-donated t-shirts bearing the names of sports teams, universities, and companies – shirts resold to them by roadside vendors.

There is no way we can ever care for everyone who shows up. What can we possibly offer to so many people?

"This is crazy!" I say to one of our Kenyan hosts. "We'll never get through them all." During a typical workday at home, I see several patients, prepare Epic notes, mark diagnoses, check billing codes, click all of the boxes, and close the charts. If I am lucky, I get through twenty people.

"We told them that the Americans would be here this week, so they showed up." He smiles. "No problem."

The ENT Clinic in Eldoret, Kenya is an exercise in controlled bedlam. The handwritten records focus on medical problems rather than billing. Scans and ultrasounds, when available, remind me of our technology from 1980, despite that it is 2014. We jam two or three patients in the same exam room with the Kenyan and US doctors, nurses, and medical students peering over each other's shoulders; there is no pretense of privacy. Patients for whom we have something to offer nod and move to the nurse's desk to add their names to the surgical schedule. Patients for whom we have nothing to offer nod and head home.

At the end of the day, I look down the hallway. There are several people who have likely been waiting since early in the morning. "They will come back tomorrow." And they do.

At home, I become annoyed when I must wait twenty minutes for an appointment; I know that patients often wait longer than that to see me. I wonder how it feels to wait hours for an opportunity – maybe the *only* opportunity – to see a specialist and then be told to return the next day or, maybe, never at all.

I became a bit more tolerant of waiting during our overseas trips. This came into focus for me on the way home from one of our first humanitarian experiences. We were returning from

El Salvador, having seen dozens of patients who had been unfailingly gracious.

At the end of the final day of the visit, the lines were still growing. My wife, Kathi, who dusted off her nursing skills for the trip, accompanied an interpreter to talk to the people lining up. "*Lo siento* (I'm sorry)," the interpreter said. "The clinic can see no more patients. The doctors and nurses must return to San Salvador now and will not be back until next year."

"That's all right," one of the women responded. "Then we will return next year, as well. Thank you for coming to help us."

The next day, we were in Houston, waiting for a connecting flight, and Kathi was telling the story of the woman standing in line to our traveling companions. Everyone shared similar experiences. As they were talking, the gate agent announced that our plane would be delayed several hours because of a major storm disrupting air traffic all along the eastern seaboard.

Immediately, an irate traveler with a sunburn strode up to the counter. "This is outrageous!" he shouted. We all looked up as he berated the agent. "We are heading back from our vacation in Mexico, and I have important meetings in the morning! I demand that you reroute us or get us on another airline! Do it now!"

The gate agent apologized and said that there were no options; *every* airline was affected by the storm. The man paced the waiting area, and we all looked up whenever he returned to the counter to register his displeasure. Finally, he announced that he was taking his family to a hotel and that the airline had better cover his bill. Off he stormed, family in tow.

"What a contrast!" Kathi noted. "Imagine if the Salvadorans who waited for us had reacted that way." We were not blind to the grinding poverty in El Salvador and had heard stories about the people's lack of opportunity, safety, services, and health care (a process Paul Farmer terms "structural violence"), but we had all noted how gracious the patients were during our one-on-one interactions.

A while after the angry man and his family had headed to their hotel, a plane arrived. We were very late getting home but did manage to sleep in our own beds.

Maybe the airline passenger's ire was more noticeable to us because we were transitioning out of a starkly different environment. As Farmer has noted, "The voices, the faces, the suffering of the sick and the poor are all around us. Can we see and hear them? Well-defended against troubling incursions of doubt, we the privileged are precisely the people most at risk of remaining oblivious, since this kind of suffering is not central to our own experience."

Global health opportunities open us to viewing life through a different lens. At every stop, the lines are long. Our memories fill with people, each one hoping that they will be rewarded with a word of hope and healing when their time of waiting is finally done.

INTERLUDE

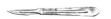

Final Words

We are what we repeatedly do.
Excellence, then, is not an act but a habit.
- Historian Will Durant

For better or worse, each of my high school English teachers was a perfectionist in their own, unique way. Each held a precise image of the perfectly crafted essay; unfortunately, these images rarely overlapped. A paper that would have garnered an "A" at the end of one school year routinely received a "C-" at the beginning of the next. Therefore, every September I found myself struggling to adopt a brand-new writing style. For the next nine months, I would master the new approach only to have it discarded and replaced again the following year. It was frustrating, but eventually I discovered that my teachers were less cranky when I turned in work that was grammatically accurate, unambiguous, and tightly crafted. That alone seemed to please all of them.

As I labored over my editing, I wondered if my teachers were just as intense and unforgiving in their private lives. Did they keep a red pen handy whenever they read a newspaper or magazine? Did they feel the urge to pick up the telephone whenever a radio announcer split an infinitive or a news anchor ended a sentence with a preposition? I suspected that they were always on-duty, even though I could not be certain.

Decades later, and long after my days of trying to please English teachers, my question is answered. A patient shares a story about an elderly relative who happened to be a retired high school English teacher. The old man was a stickler both in and out of the classroom, and his family had learned to treat the English language with respect whenever they were in his presence.

The teacher had lived a long and productive life. My patient tells me that as his death was drawing near, he was admitted to a hospice unit, spending his final days in bed too weak, even, to turn side-to-side.

One of the nurses stopped by his room. "Mr. Cooper," she said, "you look uncomfortable. Would you like to lay on your other side for a while?"

Mr. Cooper slowly and deliberately opened his eyes just wide enough to peer at her. "It's 'lie,'" he whispered. "You must say, 'Would you like to *lie* on your other side?'" The effort he expended correcting this egregious grammatical blunder overwhelmed him. He closed his eyes and groaned aloud. The family swears those were his very last words.

PART THREE

Moments of Clarity and Grace

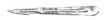

The Book

I do not at all understand the mystery of grace - only that it meets us where we are but does not leave us where it found us.
- Anne Lamott

Had Jack been born at a different time or in a different place, he might have been a character actor in the movies, a regular in the chorus on the Shakespearean stage, or a traveling troubadour. As it is, though, he is just barely bumping along at the margins, cheerful as can be.

His outward appearance is startling: a disproportionately large face and a mop of dark hair, always wild. In conversation, I have to choose which of his eyes to engage. His animated limbs are gangly and their final resting places unpredictable. His high-pitched voice does not seem to fit his long, lean body. When he folds himself into the examination room chair, his hand shoots out in greeting, an innocent smile washes over his face, and he squeaks, "Hi, Doc!" He is, safe to say, memorable.

He was sent to see me after he admitted to an urgent care physician he was having "a little trouble swallowing." When I examine his throat, I find the largest, most extensive cancer I have ever seen. His tongue, tonsil, palate, larynx, and pharyngeal wall are all replaced by a red, beefy, and overgrown malignancy.

I biopsy his throat and order some scans, which confirm the diagnosis.

His treatment options are extremely limited. With a mass so large, I am worried that he might choke to death if we don't do something soon. After a workup and discussion of his case with colleagues in the cancer center, and with Jack's permission, he is scheduled for what we assume will be a marginally effective short course of palliative radiation treatments. He will receive two large-dose treatments per week for three weeks – an approach that many centers use to treat symptoms when the goal is to relieve suffering and not to cure cancer.

Surprisingly, he has a brisk and encouraging early response even after the first two sessions. Instead of continuing on with the palliative approach, our radiation oncologist switches him to a standard curative treatment course of daily treatments for seven weeks. Although his tumor continues to melt, I assume he will never swallow again because of the large scars that will likely form as the cancer evaporates. Wrong again. He recovers steadily and resumes his previous life not long after treatment is completed. No scars, no significant adverse effects. He has a little pain that is easily controlled. His response and cure are completely unexpected, and we tell him this.

Jack recovers. At every follow-up visit, he squeaks, "You really didn't think I would make it, did you, Doc?" He always greets me warmly and thanks me profusely.

The miraculous cure holds up over time. We settle into a follow-up routine that requires less frequent visits. He calls occasionally for refills of his pain medication, but there is no uptick in the pill count, so we contact the pharmacy with authorizations. With every call, he tells my administrative assistant, who by this time is new and has never met him, what a great surgeon I am. As she relays each message, I smile, assuming that the compliment has more to do with making certain he gets timely prescription refills than any personal feelings for me.

Several years later, I receive a package from him. Inside is a used book with a torn dust jacket, bent corners, and a price tag that reads "25¢." It is a biography of Dr. Tom Dooley, published in the early 1960s. Along with the book, my patient has enclosed a handwritten note, written in pencil, thanking me for "being the best doctor I know." No other explanation. I wonder at the gesture, shake my head, and set the book aside, unread.

I recall now that I always intended to respond to the gift, but I am ashamed to say I did not. A thank-you note would have taken just a few seconds. Of course, I rationalized that he might not even receive the note because he was frequently homeless. Perhaps, though, I was uncertain of the meaning of the gift. I left note-writing for another day, perhaps hoping to eventually find the right words. Before long, preparing a response dropped entirely off my mental priority to-do list.

Winters in Wisconsin are harsh. A couple of years later, when the snow finally starts to thaw in March, some kids discover his partially submerged body in a park lagoon across the road from where he last lived. The newspaper, in a one-paragraph story, notes that his roommate reported him missing in late December. There is no further information other than that he had no known relatives.

Stunned, I pull his book from my shelf. Tom Dooley, about whom I had known very little, established a network of charity health facilities for the poor of Vietnam, Laos, and Cambodia in the 1950s. In 1960, a Gallup Poll identified him as one of America's Ten Most Admired Men. Dooley knew Albert Schweitzer, and Dooley's work is credited with inspiring the birth of the Peace Corps. When Dr. Dooley developed malignant melanoma and died in 1961 at the age of thirty-four, the world mourned his short but incredibly productive life. As I breathe in the musty pages, I wonder: *Did my patient read this book before he sent it to me? Had I really reminded him of this dynamic, virtuous, unselfish physician who improved the lives of thousands of people? Or was the book meant to inspire me to approximate Dooley's character?* I will forever ponder these questions.

The gift makes me feel unworthy and uncomfortable. I recycle the note and give the book away.

Sometime later, I run across an insight from child psychiatrist and author Robert Coles that, "the busy, capable doctor, well aware of all the burdens he must carry, and not in the least inclined to shirk his duties, may stumble badly in those small moral moments that constantly press upon him or her—the nature of a hello or good-bye, the tone of voice as a question is asked or answered, the private thoughts one has, and the effect they have on our face, our hands as they do their work, our posture, our gait."

Wow, I think. *That was me.*

I know it is far too late in coming (and I really do apologize for that) but, Jack, thanks for the book. Rest in peace, my friend.

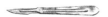

A Fullness of Uncertain Significance

Practice isn't the thing you do once you're good.
It's the thing you do that makes you good.
- Malcolm Gladwell

"Whaddya think, Doc? How bad is it? Am I gonna need more chemo and radiation? Jeez, I can't imagine going through that one more time. Be honest with me, Doc! You're the specialist. Tell me what to do." Harry fidgets in the exam chair, peppering me with questions as I wait for the latest CT scan to load onto the computer. He is pushing seventy, and his skin is weathered from years of outdoor work. His wife, Martha, looks on, notebook in lap, near tears. The scan seems to be taking longer than usual.

His tongue cancer treatment was rugged. In the months after his six-hour surgery and reconstruction, his wife mastered his feeding tube and medication schedules. He missed long stretches of work because of his postoperative radiation and chemotherapy. Despite his inherent optimism, healing took a long time.

Two years later, he still seizes every possible opportunity to credit his wife – "my rock," he calls her – for his recovery. She fills in gaps during conversations. "My memory is failing me.

Why is that?" To see him now, though, most people would be surprised that Harry has been through such an ordeal.

A few weeks ago, his throat was scratchy. "Not pain, really, but I thought things felt different, you know?" He called his primary doctor's office thinking he might need a throat culture or some antibiotics. She looked in his mouth and ordered the CT scan.

"The family doc called me a couple of days after the scan and read parts of the report to me. She sounded really worried. Doc! You have no idea how scared the wife and I have been! I haven't slept for a couple of days waiting to get in to see you."

I look through the report as I wait for the computer to finish bringing up the images. The radiologist includes phrases like "asymmetry," "fullness of uncertain significance," "probable mass," "cannot rule out recurrent cancer," "might represent metastatic nodes," and "suggest clinical correlation." Martha has underlined some of the terms and anatomical site names that they looked up on the internet.

The images finally finish loading, and I scroll through them. The oral cavity is not symmetric, an often-worrisome finding. The left side of the tongue is noticeably larger than the right. The lymph nodes are much more obvious on the left side. The structures within the neck tissues are densely scarred together. The radiologist from the other hospital, knowing nothing about our surgery, has identified many of the changes our surgery left behind without realizing that these changes were expected. I take note of a couple areas I need to focus on during the exam.

"Okay, I think I know what's going on here," I say as I wash my hands and slip on examination gloves. "Open up. Let's take a look," The tongue remnant on the left side is larger than the right, but it is soft and supple. This appears to be unchanged from his last visit. I shine my light in his mouth and throat. I press against the tissues inside the mouth and, using the fingers from both of my hands, feel the surgical scars and the tissues that lie between the lining of the mouth and the skin of the upper neck. Nothing seems to have changed over the past few months.

I check my notes from that previous visit and pull up the CT images from a scan that had been performed at our own hospital a few months ago. I compare the old scan side-by-side with the new one. Harry and Martha shift in their chairs. I recheck everything.

Nothing has changed. No new problems. Nothing worrisome at all.

"It's all good news! It is completely stable. I can explain all of the findings in the new scan based on your cancer treatment. The scan looks the same today as it did a few months ago."

"But, Doc!" Martha protests. "What about the report?" She consults her notepad. "All of those lymph nodes? How do you explain them?" She is still not convinced. "Our family doctor told me to get him in to see you right away. She is certain that his cancer had returned!"

"These nodes here are not large; they are only more noticeable because we removed the nodes from the *other* side. Same for the tongue; we removed part of the right side of the tongue and rebuilt it with the flap. That's why the left side looks bigger." I point to the computer screen images. "It's supposed to look this way." I meet their eyes, first hers then his. "Everything is fine. Absolutely fine."

I sympathize with the other doctor's anxiety. She read the radiologist's report and, reading between the lines, sensed the concern. As a family physician, she has little experience working with patients who have had uncommon operations for unusual cancers. Even if she had been pretty certain that he was cancer-free, I suspect that she would not have felt empowered to tell them not to worry. Instead, she made certain that he returned to my office as soon as possible. She did not want to overlook a new symptom or uncertain findings in a patient who is at risk for more cancer.

Of course, I can recall times when I sounded the "all clear" and the cancer returned later. More than once, I have had patients return earlier than scheduled with new cancers or worrisome symptoms. I tell people, "Do not worry," with trepidation and humility. Nevertheless, today, for this patient, at this time, I am comfortable providing reassurance. The examination and the scans are completely stable. All is well.

"Hoo, boy!" Harry slaps the arm of the exam chair. "She really had us going for a couple of days! Of course, the wife was more scared than me!" Harry winks at Martha, and she rolls her eyes. "Time to celebrate! Thanks, Doc!"

Martha shakes her head and then, for the first time, laughs.

"You're welcome." I check a couple of boxes on the computer screen, and we all sit wordlessly.

"Oh, by the way, the nurse said my blood pressure was high when I checked in today. Should I be taking something for that? What would you suggest?"

Now, I am out of my element. "Uh, you should talk to your family doctor about that. None of the medications they use these days had even been discovered when I was in medical school." Another silence. "So, get that checked. I'll see you both in a few months, okay?"

Harry eyes me as he rises from the examination chair. "So that is when you think it will recur?" He grins, and Martha pops him on the shoulder. After another chuckle, they are gone.

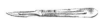

Inside Out

Life must be understood backwards;
but . . . it must be lived forward.

- Søren Kierkegaard

Bumping the door open with my right hip, I enter the operating room, water still dripping from my elbows. Toweling off my arms, I survey the patient, the equipment, and the instruments.

A stack of papers on a table next to the door catches my eye. One of the residents has taken copious notes from textbooks and journals. On a single sheet of paper, he has created a step-by-step how-to guide of today's operation from incision to closure. The list is very, very thorough. I smile and make a mental note to change up the sequence as much as possible.

I loved learning all about surgery when I was a resident! I, too, carefully summarized and underlined all of the surgical descriptions I could find. I hoped that creating those lists would give me confidence.

My attention returns to the operating room activity. I slip on my gown and gloves. While the nurse scrubs the neck skin, I make a final visual check of the patient, whose elbows and wrists have been carefully padded and tucked at his sides. A rolled-up sheet has been positioned beneath his shoulders, extending his head and fully exposing his neck. I look again to make certain that the back of his head rests gently in a sponge support. I take in the entire room, noticing the lines, cords, and tubes which connect to the patient. The sounds in the room – the hum, the beeps, the ventilator, the chatter – are all familiar and correct.

After stepping up to the table, the technologist and I place the first of the sterile towels that will cordon off the rest of the body from the operative field. We add more and more sterile coverings until only the operative site is visible. The warming blanket comes to life, and the drapes rise as heated air circulates between the patient and the overlying drapes.

The residents and a medical student join me around the table. After marking the proposed incision, I assume the familiar stance I will hold for the next two hours.

Finally, I place my hand on the patient's neck, gently manipulating the enlarged masses below the surface.

"Here," I urge. "Feel the tumors and how they sit beneath the muscles. Can you appreciate how they move in relationship with the other tissues?" The medical student wiggles the growths, simultaneously afraid of and yet fascinated by them. The older trainees move the tumors around with more self-assurance, yet I wonder what their hands are telling them.

Now, I take my turn.

I take hold of the cancer. The patient's taut neck skin below my fingers gradually becomes translucent, and the room goes silent. Soon, the muscles, arteries, veins, nerves, bones, viscera, and lymph nodes come into focus. I knead the tissues, gauging their textures and resilience, gliding the masses over the underlying structures and testing their mobility to determine if they will yield to the dissection. I work my fingers along the normal landmarks to make certain that they are not affected by the tumors. The muscles and vessels intertwine with each other and with the invasive cancer. As my mind reconstructs the scene below the skin, I visualize how the completed surgical dissection will look two hours from now, once all of the structures have been cleared of nodes, fat, and cancer, and all of the specimens have been sent to the laboratory.

The sounds in the room again reach my ears as I release my focus.

From this point, I can take hundreds of potential paths and arrive at the procedure's completion. Across the table from me, the resident who created the step-by-step list stands ready, as well. I assess his level of anxiety. His cookbook method allows for just one clear path from start to finish. I try to remember how I felt as a resident just prior to a major operation, but all I can recall is fear. For just a moment, I wonder what happened to all of those lists I so carefully created.

The team is poised. The nurse runs us through a time-out. Even after hundreds of similar procedures, I feel a twinge of doubt mixed with wonder as the case begins.

"Ready?" I have already glimpsed the surgical procedure's outcome. The knife hovers above the skin. "Let's begin."

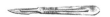

First, Do No Harm

Old age is no place for sissies.
- Bette Davis

"I want the surgery today!" Mrs. Burlingham says and then begins to cry. "I'm ninety-four years old. I'll accept any risk. Just take this thing out!"

The anesthesiologist and I exchange glances. We are standing at the foot of her cart in the pre-op area where she is being readied for surgery. Her golf ball sized tongue cancer has been growing over the past six months, and I can tell that articulation has become more difficult for her than when we first met three weeks ago. A misunderstanding about which medication to stop before surgery had her discontinue both her blood thinner (a good idea) and her blood pressure pills (not a good idea).

"I'm so close!" she says. Indeed. Her IV is in place and we are just down the hall from the operating room. She is ready for her surgery.

Everything seemed set until her nurse took her vitals. "I checked it twice," the nurse tells us. "Her blood pressure is 210 over 115."

The anesthesiologist moves into her explanation. "I'm sorry, but it's not safe to put you to sleep when your pressure is so elevated," she says. "You are at an increased risk for a stroke or heart attack. If you restart your pills, your blood pressure will probably be back in the normal range in a week or so."

"Oh, no! Oh, Doctor, I can't live with this another minute!" She buries her face in her hands and weeps.

To her it must seem simple, but there are many issues at play. There are increased anesthesia risks in the elderly. Whenever I perform surgery on an older adult, I know they are less likely to bounce back from a procedure and that their rate of complications is increased. There is a higher risk that they might end up spending time in a nursing facility. The margins of error can be razor thin. Waiting two weeks would allow her family doctor to stabilize her blood pressure and improve the odds that she will wake up safely. Despite her tears, I try to mute my emotional response; I don't want to risk a catastrophic event if we put her to sleep. Waiting is safer.

But, I think, *is there an alternative? Might I be able to safely remove the tongue cancer using only a local anesthetic?* Unfortunately, the cancer is relatively large, and it might be difficult to completely anesthetize. *What if I get the cancer halfway removed and it starts bleeding uncontrollably or she cannot tolerate lying on her back or holding her mouth open?* There is no question that, given the size and location of the cancer as well as the possibility of the case turning out to be more complex than I can anticipate before we start, I would prefer having her asleep with a breathing tube in place to prevent blood or secretions from being accidentally inhaled into her lungs. There are so many unknowns.

The possibility of performing the procedure under local continues to gnaw at me, though. During my training, older surgeons shared stories of procedures they had performed under local anesthesia for which we now routinely put people to sleep. For example, one of my mentors performed all tonsillectomies in adults under local anesthesia. To me, this seems scary and unfamiliar, but it was, at one time, the accepted technique. Old textbooks talk about big operations performed without general anesthesia.

I once saw an elderly woman who was much less robust than Mrs. Burlingham with a small, very painful tongue mass. Seeing no other options, she allowed me to remove the cancer under local anesthesia. Happily, the procedure and recovery both went very smoothly. It all comes down to weighing the risks and benefits.

I faced a similar dilemma in my own family. One day near the end of my residency training, my father called me. "What do you think we should we do?" he asked me. "The doctor says your grandmother needs surgery."

My ninety-one-year-old, bedridden grandmother was living out her final days several hundred miles away from us in a nursing home. She had severe dementia and had not recognized anyone for a decade. Over the course of a few months, one of her feet had lost all blood circulation. She was in no pain and was completely unaware that part of her leg was essentially dead. A surgeon called my father recommending that she undergo an amputation.

"Dad, what did the doctor say? Why do they want to operate?"

"Things are getting worse. If they don't take off her foot, they think that an infection might develop and then spread through her body. The infection would probably kill her."

I could not imagine that an operation would improve her

quality of life. This was no longer the energetic woman who had lived all her life on the family farm, weathering the Depression, milking cows, raising and slaughtering chickens, and watching both of her sons head to far-away wars. The woman we had known and loved had disappeared into the fog of Alzheimer's years before.

The surgeon was probably correct that an amputation would stave off an infection. We had visited her recently, though, and I was also certain that an operation would not make her feel better. She clearly did not have long to live, no matter what we decided. It seemed to me that the proposed surgery was all risk and no benefit.

I weighed the potential ethical issues, as well. If we decided to "let her go," might it appear as though we would stand to gain something from that decision? For some families, a shorter nursing home stay translates into a larger inheritance. Fortunately, her nursing home costs were covered by insurance, so that was not an issue for us. And, I wondered, why was the surgeon making the recommendation for surgery now? Was he basing it on her well-being? Or making a recommendation based strictly on the appearance of her foot?

"Dad," I said finally, "if he is only concerned about her foot, tell him no. The nursing home can make her comfortable. I don't think the surgery will make her feel any better."

My dad did not give the surgeon permission and my grandmother died – comfortably – a few weeks later.

But Mrs. Burlingham's situation is different. She is awake, alert, in pain, and able to make her own decisions. Unlike my grandmother, this woman is in otherwise good health. What should we do?

I tell Mrs. Burlingham I might be able to perform the surgery with a local anesthetic. I explain the risks as carefully as I can, and the anesthesiologist agrees to give her a little sedation – "just a touch" – for the operation. She will not be completely asleep. Mrs. Burlingham is overjoyed, and other than the blood pressure problems, she is ready for surgery.

"Okay," I tell her, "let's review things once more. If you are up to it, today is the day." The patient grips my hand and smiles. Her family members look anxious but agree, as well. Soon we are underway.

The sedation works beautifully. She barely flinches as I inject the local anesthetic all around her cancer. I don't need to modify my usual approach very much. I work as carefully and as efficiently as I can. I tie or cauterize every tiny blood vessel, working meticulously to keep blood from accumulating or dripping down her throat. The mass is large, but it comes loose from its attachments. She remains comfortable.

Soon, I make the final cut, and the mass is out. She has lost almost no blood. We place a line of stitches where the tumor had been. She goes to the recovery room, and we will watch her carefully for bleeding and swelling.

She's still groggy when I head down to talk to the family. "Things went well," I tell them. "I was able to remove all of the cancer, and she is in the recovery room. It's good news." They look as relieved as I am.

I head back upstairs and check on her. She opens her eyes and squeezes my hand. Finally, I know we made the right choice. Until that point, however, I hadn't been completely certain.

A week later, Mrs. Burlingham returns to the office, tearfully thanking me for the operation. "I'm pain-free!" she says. "I felt better right away. I never even needed any pain medicine after I went home." Her family confirms this. She grabs my hand. "Doctor, you must always listen to old people! We know what we're talking about!"

Every surgeon is asked, "Doctor, if she was your grandmother, what would you do?" Surgical decision-making is best based on evidence, but choosing a particular option for any individual person still boils down to an imperfect choice. We gather information, then weigh the risks and the benefits. Though the decision for my own grandmother was different from that for Mrs. Burlingham, I stand by them both.

Hippocrates instructed us thus: *"Primum non nocere"* – *"First, do no harm."* For Mrs. Burlingham, and for my grandmother, things turned out as they were supposed to.

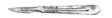

Far from Home

Trust your instinct to the end, though you can render no reason.
- Ralph Waldo Emerson

We are in the middle of an all-day ENT screening clinic in Eldoret, Kenya at the Moi Teaching and Referral Hospital. The local ENT physicians have scheduled about one hundred patients to see our American team and be evaluated for surgery during our visit. We have already seen several people with baseball-sized tumors in their parotids, thyroids, or necks. The surgical schedule for the next few days is filling quickly.

A thirteen-year-old boy sits in the exam chair. His father sits next to him. Henry, my wonderful Kenyan ENT colleague, hands me an X-ray with some blurry images.

"This boy's neck mass has been growing steadily for the past two years. We were able to get a CT scan at another hospital in town since our scanner has been broken for the past year. The radiologist believes he has a glomus vagale tumor." Henry looks at me. "Do you agree?"

I hold the scan up to the light streaming through a nearby window to illuminate the images. The mass is very large – filling much of the side of his neck – and it displaces the carotid artery that carries blood from the heart to the brain. The mass is bright white on the scan, confirming its very rich blood supply, and extends from the level of the jawline to the collarbone. The diagnosis is likely correct, although it could be a different kind of tumor. At home, I would lean on my radiologist, trusting her to confirm the diagnosis. *This probably is a glomus vagale tumor,* I think to myself, *but what if it isn't?* I need to be extra vigilant this far from home.

"How would you care for this in the United States?" Henry asks me.

"Well," I say, "we would probably get some additional scans and order laboratory tests to make certain he doesn't have a condition that runs in his family or one that might cause severe blood pressure problems in surgery. And we would send him to the specialized interventional radiologists and ask them to squirt some material into the mass before an operation to cut down on the bleeding. Bleeding during this kind of surgery can be very dangerous, even fatal."

"Those things aren't available here," Henry tells me. "He would have to go to Nairobi. Four hours away. Oh, and I should mention that we do not have any blood transfusions available for surgery." Henry smiles at me. "Can't we just remove it?"

"It's not a simple case," I protest. I have goals for the surgical procedures we schedule during these trips: every operation should leave the patient better off, expand the skill set of the local surgeons, and reside reasonably close to my personal surgical "comfort zone." This case, with its less-than-certain diagnosis and potential for bleeding and significant complications, makes me anxious.

"The mass is growing," Henry reminds me after talking to the boy's father in Kiswahili. The boy sits quietly in the chair, glancing back and forth between his father and Henry. His face is placid.

The goal of an operation would be to completely remove the tumor with as little blood loss as possible while saving the maze of anatomic structures plastered to its surface. Bluntly, we warn them that surgery might cause a stroke or paralysis of nerves that control the tongue, voice box, and shoulder. He could die. "What happens if we don't operate?" the father asks. The mass will enlarge and become more entangled. There are risks both ways. I suspect they will decline the operation.

The boy looks peaceful. The father speaks quietly to Henry, who relays his words. "They want you to go ahead. Shall we schedule for Monday?"

Hoo-boy.

Working in Kenya sometimes reminds me of earlier times in my training.

When I was a junior resident, rotating through the VA Hospital and at the Milwaukee County Medical Complex in the early 1980s, there were days when I felt very much alone. Sometimes, we cared for patients without supervision. If we could find medical records, they were often illegible. X-rays and scans were hard to locate. The available technology and techniques would now seem archaic. It was all we knew at the time, but I shudder to think of the disasters we barely avoided. As we contemplate this boy's operation, I have a flashback or two.

"Are you certain that they really understand the risks?"

Henry assures me that they do.

Over the next few days, I mentally rehearse the procedure. *What tricks can we employ? What old pearls can I conjure? What would some of my mentors have done?* Over the weekend,

I mention to Susan, one of the other surgeons on the team, that the case is making me nervous. "Yeah," she says, "I wondered why you put that one on the schedule."

I debate canceling. I think about the boy and his father. I alternate between confidence that we will be able to safely remove the mass and anxiety about the decision to operate. *This isn't straightforward,* I think to myself. *If we don't take it out now, it will be an even greater challenge next year or the year after that.* Then I think, *But is that reason enough?*

On Monday, I stand across the operating table from Henry and Susan. My son, David, a fourth-year medical student at the time, is holding retractors.

As predicted, the procedure is difficult. We immediately face a tangle of blood vessels ranging from fragile, corkscrew-like veins to large, pulsating arteries. There are diffuse, dense attachments to the surrounding tissues and direct involvement of the vagus nerve (which controls movement of the vocal cords, among other functions). Every move requires planning and care as we dissect the mass away from the major blood vessels and critical structures.

The mass begins to ooze, a little at first and then disturbingly. I try to cauterize the bleeding points, but it only makes things worse. I hold pressure on the mass. This helps, but every time I release the pressure, the blood begins flowing again. "Let's just keep going," I say. As long as I keep pressure on the mass, things remain under control. We press on.

Time telescopes. My whole body is on high alert. Everything is in sharp focus.

After two hours, thanks to great colleagues, caution, and good fortune, the mass is removed. The bleeding stops. Normal time resumes, and I realize that the temperature in the operating room is in the mid-eighties. I am drenched in sweat. We close the wound and send the patient to the recovery room where he wakes up quickly. He seems fine.

The next day, we make morning rounds. The young boy is sitting in bed, not quite smiling but on the mend. The mass is in the laboratory, and hopefully we will get a final pathology report in about a month. As I look at his neck wound, I realize that I am still reeling a bit from the case and am incredibly grateful that he is alive and recovering nicely. I feel alive, as well.

I wave to the boy and he smiles. As soon as we finish making rounds, we all head to the operating room for another day of surgery.

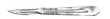

Remembering Moments

We do not remember days, we remember moments.
- Cesare Pavese

My colleague bursts through the door of my operating room. "A plane! A plane just crashed into the World Trade Center."

I look up from where I am standing next to the operating table. My resident and I have been removing a malignant mass from my patient's neck. The surgery has just started, but the scars from another surgeon's biopsy have made the initial steps of the dissection tricky.

"What?"

"A plane. I was in the OR lounge and the news switched to New York. A plane just crashed into the World Trade Center."

I stare at him. I recheck the surgical field and put pressure on the wound.

"So, what are they saying? What's going on?"

"They don't know. My God. It's awful."

He leaves, and we go back to work. The resident and I tease out the anatomy, peeling the skin from the underlying muscles, finding the jugular vein, and preserving the nerves to the tongue and the shoulder. We dissect the lymph nodes away from the surrounding tissues deep in the wound.

The door bursts open. "Another plane. This one crashed into the other tower."

"What?"

"They're replaying the videos over and over. The first tower is on fire. Then there's the other plane."

He runs out again.

We lift out some of the nodes, clearing them from the carotid artery. I can feel the patient's blood flowing from his heart to his brain through its wall.

The door opens again. "Bush was just on TV. He says it's terrorists."

I close my eyes. "Please stop. Please don't come in with any more news reports."

He pauses. "Okay, sure." Then he runs out.

We wrap up the surgery, tie off a few small blood vessels, and close the wound. It is deadly quiet. None of us in the room have any idea what is going on, but we sense it is bad. I linger as the patient wakes up. We wheel him to the recovery room.

Someone stops me in the hallway. "The first tower collapsed."

I walk to the lounge to watch with the others, then head down to the family center to talk to my patient's wife. She is watching the news along with everyone else. We step into a private consultation room so I can review her husband's surgery. We return to the waiting area where I stare at the television with her for a few minutes. The scenes of smoke billowing from the towers and the slow-motion impact of the second plane play over and over.

Everyone in the hospital looks dazed. News reports flash about a plane crashing into the Pentagon. Another plane reportedly crashes in Pennsylvania.

I wonder: *Were any of my New York friends killed? Will New York and Washington DC hospitals be overwhelmed? Many of my partners are at a meeting in Denver. Are they okay?* Flights are being cancelled and all of the airports are closed. *How will they get home? Are more attacks imminent? Are we all in danger?*

I walk back to the recovery room where my patient is waking up. I tell him that the surgery went well. He smiles and dozes off. He went to sleep in one world and will awaken in another.

Despite humankind's overwhelming capacity for kindness and compassion, we seem bent on senseless, self-inflicted tragedy. The numbers of people killed during wars and atrocities are incomprehensible. 750,000 died during the American Civil War. Approximately 85,000,000 died over the course of WWII, including the single-day death tolls of 1,177 at Pearl Harbor, 145,000 in Dresden, and 60,000 at Hiroshima. Millions have died in wars of which we have never heard and about which we never studied in school. The death tolls from slavery, racism, and brutality cannot be measured.

Survivors beg us to remember the stories, but their voices soon fade. Nineteenth century Americans were exhorted to, "Remember the Alamo!" and, "Remember the Maine!" during our wars with Mexico and Spain. The survivors of those cataclysmic events – and many others – are long gone. Their appeals no longer stir our emotions. After each moment of outrage, our collective and personal sense of innocence and the illusion of normalcy returns. Our hands return to our daily tasks. We turn away and forget.

Still, I was shaken hard that morning in September 2001. I will never understand why 3,000 people were killed that day in New York, at the Pentagon, and in a farm field in Shanksville, Pennsylvania. I mourn the hundreds of first responders and cleanup workers who were sickened or died. I despair at the subsequent thousands of dead civilians and soldiers and the millions of refugees. The gnawing emptiness in my gut during the weeks that followed mirrored the emptiness of the skies devoid of planes. Yet, the aftershocks faded. Soon, even when I tried, I could no longer evoke the depths of despair that were once so real.

For several years, the patient on whom I operated the morning the towers fell continued to come for follow-up visits. I was happy to see him. I would examine his neck and make certain his cancer had been controlled. We always spent part of the appointment reliving our shared, indelible experience.

"Do you remember?" we would ask each other.

"Yes, I do," we would respond.

Eventually, though, there was no need for him to return. No more annual visits. "Let me know if things change," I said.

He shook my hand. "I won't forget that day," he said.

"Me, either," I replied. Yet, I know now, I had already begun the process of forgetting.

The fading passion, I am certain, protects us from being locked into permanent states of grief and anger. 9/11, as well as all the shocking events that have since rocked our lives and our society, aroused outrage and grief. Each has evoked powerful emotions and calls to action. With each event, new leaders rise and inspire us to be part of the change. The events and names remain alive if we amplify the stories. We pledge to stay engaged.

9/11 remains one of my communal "Where were you?" moments. Most of the medical students with whom I now work were in grade school the day that the attacks occurred. The act of telling this story again is my way of keeping a memory of that day – and the passions it engendered in me – alive.

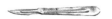

Scars

To be trusted is a greater compliment than to be loved.

- George MacDonald

I am operating in Kenya and, as we adjust the patient's position on the surgical table, I spot some short, vertical scars on the front of her neck. The parallel slashes sit directly over her enlarged thyroid – a goiter – and appear to have been deliberately placed. There are two sets of scratches, one set on either side of the neck, nearly identical in length and evenly spaced. I rub my finger across the marks; they are superficial and do not extend deeply into the underlying tissues. The scars are small quotation marks on the otherwise smooth, taut skin of the young African woman.

My Kenyan colleague, Henry, notices my interest.

"Those are tribal," he tells me.

"What do they represent?" I ask.

"They are not ceremonial markings. No, those were made by a folk healer. The healer cuts in the skin and puts medicines and herbs under the surface to make the goiter go away."

"Does it work?"

He looks at me and smiles. "Well, no. But they try, anyway."

I am assisting two of the Kenyan surgeons as they perfect their thyroidectomy skills. Kenya has a high proportion of people with symptomatic goiters, many of which cause problems with breathing or swallowing. The surgery to remove the thyroid is usually straightforward, but there are some tricks that we can share. In sub-Saharan Africa, skilled thyroid surgeons can stay very busy.

Soon, everything is ready. The neck – along with the scars – is scrubbed and draped. We are underway.

We create a horizontal incision over the lower neck and raise the skin off of the tissues to expose the thyroid gland beneath the surface. Back in the States, we would remove both sides of the gland because both lobes are enlarged and abnormal. That is not always true here.

"I talked to her when we met in the clinic," Henry tells me. "She cannot afford to purchase thyroid medication if we remove her entire gland. We need to save as much as possible."

We remove the left lobe entirely because it is pushing her windpipe far to the side and causing symptoms. On the right side, we work to save as much normal tissue as possible.

The procedure goes well. The goiter would be considered colossal at home but is fairly typical here. We finish the procedure and close the wound, returning the neck skin to its place. It is one of fourteen thyroidectomies the surgeons and I will share over the course of my month in Kenya.

We take the drapes down and prepare to move her to a cart. "Look," I say, "the little vertical scars are still there."

"Yes," responds Henry, "but now she now has a new horizontal scar, as well."

She has seen two sets of healers to get rid of the enlarged thyroid. Both the folk healer and our surgical team gave her recommendations. Now, at last, the mass is gone.

She wakes up, and we stop by the ward later to see how she is doing. The next morning, she is grateful and ready to begin the journey home. She is breathing better, and the neck skin is a little swollen.

She should heal quickly, but the scars – those small vertical marks and the longer horizontal incision – signify two moments when she placed her trust in others. Those scars will remain.

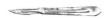

Across the Divide

Proximity and closeness are not the same.
- Thi Bui

I draw back the curtain and step within. Mr. Buchanan is lying on the bed, chatting with one of the pre-op nurses. "Ah," he says, grinning at me, "my surgeon has arrived! You remember my daughter, Jessica, don't you? And this is Emma!" He is a robust, engaging seventy-one-year-old man whose personality fills the room. Jessica smiles. She sits with one hand on the side rail of his bed. Emma, who is about five, looks intently at me from her mother's lap.

"Good morning, everybody! All set? I need to mark the surgical site." The cubicle is busy. While the nurse enters Mr. Buchanan's vitals on the computer, the anesthesiologist explains the process for putting him to sleep. I pick up a felt-tip marker and write the word "yes" and my initials on the side of his neck where the cancer gently distorts the contour of his cheek. I recall his CT scan and biopsy report. We already know this mass is a cancer. As I mark the skin, my fingers confirm its texture, size, and density. I try to imagine what we will find in the OR. Our goal today will be to remove the cancer and the nearby lymph nodes completely.

I recap the marker and step back. "So, tell me how you've been doing," I say. His smile widens.

"I'm fine, Doc," he says. "Really good. Did you get a good night's sleep?"

I shake my hands, pretending I have developed a spectacular tremor. "Once I finally went to bed, I slept okay. I was up most of the night reading about your surgical procedure and weeping uncontrollably."

He laughs. "You kill me, Doc!"

"We'll try not to," I promise. Jessica groans and shakes her head.

I grow a bit more serious and look back and forth between them. "Anything at all you want to ask about? Anything?"

He shakes his head and looks at Jessica. She shakes her head, as well.

"Nah. We've talked about the surgery and we're ready. Take good care of me, okay? And keep Jessica posted, will ya'?"

"Of course, we will." I turn to Jessica. "I'll come and find you in the family center when we're done." I smile at Emma. "And how about you, Emma?" I ask. "Any questions?" She buries her face in her mother's arm. "Oh, I'll bet you are always this quiet and shy, right?"

Jessica tries unsuccessfully to coax Emma to look up. "Not a chance! C'mon, Emma, say hello."

Emma's face stays buried in her mother's sleeve, and I remember how my own children reacted to strangers when they were young. "That's okay, Emma. I'll come and find you later, too, okay?"

Without looking up, Emma's head bobs up and down.

Soon, we are in the operating room. My resident and I work for four hours, steadily freeing up the cancer that has grown in Mr. Buchanan's cheek and spread to the lymph nodes in his neck. Although this is a procedure I have done often, the surgery turns out to be quite difficult, and the cancer is close to several important structures and nerves. We finally tease it out and send it to the laboratory. We recheck the entire surgical field, place a drain, and sew up the wound. The anesthesiologist awakens him from sleep, and we move him onto a rolling cart for his trip to the recovery room.

I head to the family center and find Jessica and Emma. "He did well," I tell them, "and we met all of our goals." I draw a diagram of the surgery. Jessica takes notes as we talk, and she asks about what to expect in the coming weeks. "The report will come back from the pathologist in three or four days. After we get the report, we will be able to make recommendations on whether he needs more treatment. In any case," I say, "he should be ready to go home tomorrow."

Jessica asks a few more questions about wound care and diet. She sighs. "He will probably play golf tomorrow afternoon no matter what you say." I shrug. She folds my diagram and tucks it into her notebook.

All the time Jessica and I have been talking, Emma has been concentrating intently on her coloring book. I tap her on the arm. "What are you working on?" I ask.

She looks up at me very seriously and turns the page to show me. It is a scene from the movie *Frozen*. "I'm coloring a picture of Elsa and Anna. It's for Grandpa."

"Wow!" I say. "That's beautiful! He will love it." I pause, and she starts coloring again. "So, Emma, your mommy got to ask questions. Do you have any?"

Without looking up, she says, "Will Grandpa be all right?"

She has asked the simplest – yet most profound – question of all.

As I watch her color, I remember an essay by poet and farmer Wendell Berry entitled "Health is Membership." Berry describes a pivotal time in his own life. His brother was in critical condition after having undergone emergency heart surgery. During the days following the operation, Berry sensed that the family was living at the interface of two worlds separated by an unbridgeable chasm.

On the patient's side of the chasm was the world of love consisting of friends, family, and community. On the health care side of the chasm was the world of efficiency, machinery, and statistical probability. Berry notes, "the world of love meets the world of efficiency . . . or, rather, these two worlds come together in the hospital but do not meet."

The family center – along with other hospital locations like the cancer clinic and the bedside – are places where the worlds of love and efficiency press hard upon one another. On this day, my feet are firmly planted in the world of efficiency, while Emma and her mother inhabit the world of love.

As I grew into this profession, my patients taught me that I could best fulfill my calling as a healer when I recognized the presence of the chasm. Emma's question is a difficult one, and she deserves an answer. Her grandpa's cancer is dangerous, and I honestly do not know how he will do. I do know, however, that we will all be taking this journey together.

"Emma," I say, "your grandpa is doing great, and we will care for him in every way we possibly can. Will you help us?"

She reaches for another crayon and nods.

I look across the chasm. On this day, I believe I can see Jessica and Emma from where I stand.

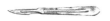

Learning

We do not exist for ourselves.
- Thomas Merton

An interlibrary loan item I had requested is ready for me to pick up, so I stop by the circulation desk. After the librarian checks my ID, she heads off to retrieve my book. I lean against the counter to wait.

The medical school library is humming quietly as medical students tap on their laptops, pore over textbooks, and review lecture notes, shielding their eyes as they try to shut out distractions. Two lean together across a table to confer about the materials in front of them. A student digs in her backpack and retrieves a pile of handouts. She adjusts her earbuds, arranges her notes carefully, and rests her elbows on the table, pressing her fingertips firmly into her forehead near the hairline. Before long, she is reading intently. No one else seems to notice the young woman nearby, half-sitting on a stool at an open computer terminal.

She stares at the computer screen, scanning page after page. She scrolls through documents, stopping abruptly to copy intently into one of the wire-bound spiral notebooks on the counter in front of her. She pulls a highlighter out of the pocket of her jeans to mark what she has written. She pushes her unruly shoulder-length brown hair away from her face, hooking her little finger around a few strands plastered to the corner of her mouth, then retrieves the elastic band from her wrist to gather her hair into a ponytail. Her eyes rarely leave the screen. Her right hand darts alternately from the notebook to the keyboard to the mouse.

Her left hand gently and methodically pushes and pulls the handle of a worn, oversized child stroller. A girl, perhaps about five years old, lies propped in the seat, her head buffered by an array of pillows and foam. The girl wears a pink pullover sweatshirt and pants, ankle socks, and unscuffed white shoes. A drop of saliva collects on her lips. A silastic tube pokes out from below her shirt. Her thin, neatly trimmed auburn hair frames her face, and her unfocused eyes gaze at the ceiling from below the clean line of her bangs.

The stroller moves back and forth. The girl's hand, suspended in midair above her chest, sways limply in rhythm with the stroller. Her breathing is steady and quiet. The woman scans the computer screen and types with one hand.

Suddenly, the girl cries out. Her face contorts, and her arm flails to the side. She emits a grunting, forlorn, agonized squeal followed by a series of weak, uncontrolled gasps. The woman pulls the stroller close, cocking her head as she looks inside. A pink stuffed kitten has toppled and now leans against the girl's leg. The woman gently rights the toy and sets it back in place. She speaks quietly as she smooths the girl's hair. "Everything's okay, sweetie," she says. "Mommy's here. Look how pretty you are." She presses a washcloth against the corner of the girl's mouth. The girl's breathing settles.

The medical student has looked up from her notes. Her chin rests on the palm of her hand as she watches. The woman's attention has shifted back to the computer screen, and she now rolls the stroller back and forth with her foot. She sets aside one notebook and presses the cover shut. She opens another notebook, grasps her pen, and stares at the screen.

"Here's your book," says the librarian to me. I turn to her and smile. "It's due back in two weeks."

"Thanks," I say. I make a mental note of the due date and take a final look around.

The expressionless child blinks, arm again swaying with the movement. The student exhales, rubs her eyes, and repositions her laptop, scrolling down the screen until she finds her place.

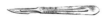

Cut Here

I was a neophyte in another world.
- Jean-Paul Sartre

The jugular vein bulges blue and taut as I dissect the enlarged lymph nodes away from its surface. A hole in the translucent vessel wall would fill the surgical field with blood and the room with frantic activity.

Today is the first day of the rotation with the new medical students. Eva, a junior student, is standing at the operating room table with me and two of our residents. This is her very first time watching surgery. I try to imagine what she is thinking. She might be watching the blood course through the jugular vein on its way from the brain back to the heart. Small eddies are visible. She might be thinking back to her college physics courses and realizing that the turbulence she notices follows a defined set of mathematical equations. Pushing on the vein would change the patterns.

Eva stands on an elevated platform to watch the surgery, mostly over the shoulder of the junior resident. Some of her medical school classmates calculate how many tuition dollars they spend for each activity of the day; at $52,000 per year and about eighty hours per week, it works out to about $14 per hour, so this three-hour operation will cost her about $42 in tuition. Her sterile gown is as clean as it was when she was tied into it about an hour ago. Her sterile gloves are bloodless. She stretches to see as we point out the anatomy and the resident describes what we are doing.

Eva watches as we work. She has had a long journey to get to this day. I have asked her about where she is from and where she went to school. She graduated with honors in Biology from a large Midwestern university after finishing at the top of her high school class. From over 8,000 applicants, she was one of about 200 students accepted into her medical school class. During the first two years, she spent countless hours studying everything from neuroscience and biochemistry to pharmacology and anatomy. It was like taking all of the toughest college courses simultaneously. She is likely accumulating educational debt at a frightening pace.

Life is more than studying, of course. I ask about her family. Her fiancée is in graduate school. Her parents live several hours away. She can't wait to get home for the holidays.

Now that she is in the third of four years of medical school, she is anxious about picking a specialty. Everything has been interesting thus far, although she thinks she would like to be a pediatrician. She loves kids, and the residents she worked with at Children's seemed happy. She looks around the room. Maybe she is thinking she might like surgery.

I continue to strip nodes and fat away from the veins and discover a small branch where it joins the jugular. This branch will need to be cut away from the main vein in order to free up the enlarged lymph nodes.

"Let's take this vein," I tell the resident. "Two clamps, please." The scrub tech hands the resident and me each a hemostat. We clamp the vein. "Tenotomy scissors." The resident cuts the small vein, and the edges separate. Eva watches as we use a piece of gauze to push against the tissues, freeing the jugular vein from the surrounding nerves and lymph nodes.

"3-0 silk ties." I lift the handle of the clamp into the air as the resident passes a piece of silk around it. I drop my wrist, pointing the tips of the clamp up as the resident throws three knots, tying off the small vein between the tip of the clamp and the jugular vein. I pass the hemostat to the tech and we repeat the process, tying off the other end of the vein.

"Okay, suture scissors to Eva," I say. She straightens up a bit as the junior resident slides to his right so she can reach the operating table. Eva reaches toward the scrub tech who places the scissors into her hand. "Cut them short," I tell her.

Eva squints as she aims the tips of the scissors toward the suture. She opens the gap between the blades.

"Just use the tips," the resident warns. "You don't want to nick the vein hiding behind the suture."

Eva withdraws the scissors and closes the blades until there is barely space between them. She moves the blades forward and engages the vertical twin strands of silk being held taut by the resident. She slides the scissors down the suture toward the knot next to the vein.

"Okay, a little shorter. Shorter, still. That's good. Cut."

Eva squeezes the scissors together. One of the two strands of silk cuts. The other frays a bit but remains intact. She opens the scissors again, pushes harder, and closes the blades again, this time cutting the suture. The frayed strand is longer than the other.

"That's okay." I aim my headlight at the knot. "Here, give

me the scissors for a second." Eva yields them, and I grab the uneven strand with forceps and trim it cleanly. "There." I hand the scissors back to Eva. "Now cut the other suture."

Eva cuts the second suture near the knot without incident. The surgery continues. There are several more opportunities to cut. With each one, she does fine, although she does display a fine tremor. "You're doing great, Eva," says one of the residents. "Nice job for your first day in the OR."

When it is time to close the wound, one of the residents offers to help guide her through placing a couple of the below-the-surface stitches that will hold the skin together. She carefully slides the needle through the muscle and fat beneath the skin and ties the knots with a surgical instrument. "I watched a video about this last night, but it is harder in real life," she says. She is tentative but places the stitches accurately. "Sorry I'm taking so long."

"You're doing fine," says the resident.

After a couple more stitches, she asks him to take over. "Show me some tricks," she says.

A few minutes later, the patient is wheeled from the OR to the recovery room. I run into Eva later in the day at a conference. "Did you enjoy your day? What surprised you most?" I ask her.

She thinks for a second. "I guess I was surprised by how different things seem in the OR compared to the rest of the world," she replies. "I mean, I've been cutting with scissors since kindergarten and sewing clothes since I was ten. Yet, this all seemed so new and scary."

"True enough," I say. "A lot of things in medicine must be relearned from scratch."

"It was really interesting," she says, "but I can't imagine how a person becomes a surgeon. There are so many things to learn."

She is correct that there are many technical things to master. "But," I respond, "it's more than learning to do procedures. Being an expert surgeon involves knowing when *not* to operate just as much as when or how to operate. That takes time. Do you think you would like to be a surgeon?"

"Maybe. Gosh! I don't know. I can't imagine how I will decide on a specialty!" she says. "I'll keep it on my list for now."

Eva developed more confidence in the operating room over the course of her rotation, and I continued to encourage her to consider becoming a surgeon. She did find her calling. Thanks in part, I'm sure, to my skillful teaching, Eva ultimately chose her specialty. She is now happily working . . . as a pediatrician.

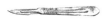

Uncertain Experts

*An expert is a person who has made all the mistakes
that can be made in a very narrow field.*
- Niels Bohr

Five experienced, well-published, and widely respected head and neck cancer surgeons are sharing the dais at the national medical meeting to explore the topic "Can We Be Better?" The panel represents a spectrum of experts from around North America who have served as program leaders, department chairs, and deans. The audience knows these people as confident surgeons who possess a wide breadth of experience. They are smart and gifted. We would trust any one of them to care for a family member.

"So," intones the moderator, who is an even *more* prominent surgeon, as he advances his PowerPoint presentation, "our panelists struggled a bit with that last case, don't you think?" The audience chuckles. The cases presented thus far have offered no clear-cut choices. "Well, why don't I make this next one even more difficult for them?"

The panelists spend an hour working through discussions of patients who have undergone extensive surgical procedures and have received radiation therapy and chemotherapy, only to have their cancers return. For some there are viable options. For others, there are no textbook answers.

"Oh, boy. That's a recurrence after treatment? Wow. I wouldn't have much to offer this man," says one of the experts.

"How about immunotherapy?" asks the moderator. "We're routinely testing the recurrent tumors for molecular targets now. Some of the patients get durable responses."

"The data are getting better, but not everyone is a candidate," says one of the panelists. "For some, the research says it extends life by only a few weeks, and the drugs cost over $10,000 per month."

One of the panelists leans to say something to another panelist, perhaps whispering he would offer it anyway.

"We have to keep in mind that about one-quarter of lifetime medical expenses occur in the final year of life," notes another.

And so it goes. Back and forth with no textbook answers. The panelists gamely quote research and recall patients who have done well and have done poorly. They suggest palliative care, hospice referrals, and comfort measures. They discuss costs. They review the principles of shared decision-making. They acknowledge that, at some point, further active treatment is always futile. As I listen, I nod. After having been in practice for many years, I share their belief that this can be a difficult, ambiguous specialty and that our options are often imperfect.

"And what if he was in his eighties instead of being in his fifties?" asks the moderator. "Would you change your mind based on his age?"

The panelists glance at each other and groan. "It depends," they say.

I look around the room and nod to one of my colleagues who practices on the East Coast. Those of us in the audience understand that the requisite skills to care for these difficult patients does not come easily, even to these world-class experts. Their abilities and judgement have accumulated slowly and in layers over the course of long and thoughtful careers.

Then one of the surgeons on the panel says this: "My worst nightmare would be to have all of my head and neck cancer patients come back from the grave to visit me."

I am shocked to hear him say this. I expect the room to gasp, but there is no sound.

I think I know what he means. When things go well, our patients live long and functional lives. When things go badly, though, the final weeks and months can be horrible for both patient and family. Although we don't talk much about it, we surgeons grieve as well, although we realize our suffering pales when compared to what the family experiences. Even when we have established solid relationships and have compassionately helped patients transition through the stages that approach the end of life, we often feel as though we have failed them.

I glance over my shoulder to check for reactions from the back rows of the conference room. These are the youngest members of the crowd, the medical students and residents who are at the beginning of their journeys. Not too many annual meetings ago, I was back there, wondering where my career would take me. The younger members of the audience are filled with anticipation and questions. What must they be thinking, watching these senior surgeons who appear to be struggling with patient care decisions despite decades of experience? If these world-famous surgeons nearing the ends of their careers remain anxious and uncertain about how best to care for difficult patients, why would these young physicians ever want to select this field of practice?

Over the years, some memorable patient encounters, welcoming families, and serendipitous moments directed my footsteps. I look back and see the connection between those days and now. I still experience anxiety more than I like to admit, although those anxious moments let me know I am still alive.

Intentionally pursuing a career that includes life-and-death decisions, ambiguity, and stressful, difficult discussions carries both risk and reward. Some of the students and residents in the back of the auditorium will, in fact, be drawn to the flame. All I know for certain is that their careers will evolve by the time they find themselves as the experts in a profession that will always be uncertain.

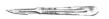

Comfort

We are in community each time we find a place where we belong.
- Peter F. Block

His clothes hang too loosely from his thin frame, but his hair is neatly combed. He dabs the corner of his lip, mopping the accumulating saliva. He has difficulty forming words, as though there is something large occupying space inside of his mouth.

I ask about his life. He lives alone and never goes out. He was a shoe salesman at a big-name local department store that went out of business years ago. He found another job selling shoes for a while but is now retired. By his own admission, he rarely strays far from his familiar neighborhood several miles from our campus.

His oral cavity pain finally sent him to a dentist down the street from his apartment building. I imagine that the dentist was shocked when she looked in his mouth. She told him that he needed to make an appointment in the head and neck clinic. Now he is here.

He speaks deliberately. "I believe that there is a problem with one of my teeth," he says. "The dentist said I should come here for help."

He does, indeed, have a problem, but it is more than just

his teeth. He cannot open his mouth fully because a huge, destructive cancer has invaded his tongue and lower jaw. It has been growing for a long time.

"When did this start?"

"The tooth began to bother me at least a year ago. It has made it hard to eat."

"How much do you think you weighed before it started to hurt?" I ask.

He shrugs. "160, last time I checked."

I look at the chart. "You weigh 115 today."

His eyes widen with surprise. Because he has never been to a doctor before, I have no idea if he has other medical problems. I grab a headlight and look in his mouth, trying to get a sense of what the mass involves. He has a neck mass that is likely a lymph node full of cancer. I steer the conversation from his dental issues to the more pressing problem. As I talk about the cancer, his eyes become glazed. He has stopped listening.

This would be a lot easier if he had someone here with him, I think. We will need help with his care. "Do you live with anyone?" I ask. "Do you have family nearby?"

He stares at his hands. "No one in town. I have a brother who lives somewhere out west. I haven't talked to him for a while. Years, actually."

As far as I can tell, he is completely adrift in the world. The touchstones of his life – his neighborhood, any friends, his brother, his former life as a shoe salesman, any familiar thing on which he might depend – are far, far away. He came to us with what he thought was a problem tooth; now, we have plunged him into a frightening and incomprehensible world, giving him a fearsome diagnosis and unknowable challenges.

Even as I promise that we will help him, he shrivels into the examination chair. I cut the discussion short, planning to go into more of the specifics at the next visit.

We will cover the details, I think to myself, *if he returns.*

Over the years, I have seen people so stunned by a diagnosis that they decided against receiving any care. I watch as my new patient appears to retreat into his shell, clasping his hands and staring at the floor. The appointment is nearing an end, and I still have no idea of how to open the door the tiniest bit. I pause.

"Rockports," he says.

"Huh?"

"Your shoes, Doctor. They're Rockports."

I look down and smile. Sure enough, I am wearing my black Rockport dress shoes today. "You're right," I reply. "I love 'em. Really comfortable."

"Great shoes." He nods and looks at me. "They practically sell themselves. Good choice."

We talk about shoes for a while then, "How about this?" I offer. "We'll complete the workup here, but let's see if we can arrange treatment at a hospital closer to your apartment. Would that help?"

He brightens. "That would be great. I am completely lost whenever I come to this part of town. It's too hard."

A few phone calls later and his treatment is arranged. I am not surprised when he returns as planned later in the week and completes all of his testing. And when he returns for a follow-up, I make certain I am wearing the shoes that provided us with our initial opportunity to connect.

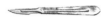

Prepared

The soul should always stand ajar,
ready to welcome the ecstatic experience.
- Emily Dickinson

Thora is nearing the end of a long and interesting life. Her birth was announced on the party line of her rural community's first telephone system. She graduated with a degree in Home Economics in the 1930s and worked for a meat packing company, teaching housewives about food safety and testing recipes during and after World War II. She wrote cookbooks, nurtured friendships, volunteered incessantly, and raised a family. Her death, which will arrive soon, will be shared via cell phone and mourned on Facebook.

She was admitted to the hospital after a slow, uneventful decline. "Failure to thrive," we physicians call it. She forgets to eat breakfast and doesn't know if her family has come to visit. Her stamina is gone, and she is no longer interested in the newspaper or the world around her. She does not care that the baseball season is nearly complete and that her beloved Chicago Cubs are, once again, well out of the running. For her family and her medical caregivers, it is a time of sadness and farewell, but at ninety-five, not unexpected.

Early one afternoon late in September, I stop by her room. She is dozing when I sit down and take her hand.

"It's so good to see you," she says as she awakens. "Are you working hard today? Lots of patients in surgery?"

"No, it's Sunday. No work today."

She smiles and closes her eyes again. Her pale skin matches her faded nightgown. Her white hair, usually well-kempt, is matted to her forehead. The TV is on but muted.

On her bedside table sits her Bible – a worn companion that has been patched back together over the years with clear contact paper. Some get-well cards are stacked next to the water pitcher. A hospital-issued toothbrush, still in its wrapper, lies next to a travel-size tube of toothpaste.

Suddenly, she opens her eyes, furrows her brow, and looks at me intently. Her thin fingers tighten around mine. I am startled. "What is it?" I ask. "Are you having pain?"

She squeezes my hand. "No, no, I'm fine. But tell me," she says. "I was wondering. Do you think I will die today?"

Her question freezes me in place. Not infrequently, a cancer patient will ask me to estimate how long they have left, and, in those instances, I try to provide them with a realistic range of weeks or months, knowing that I will usually be wrong. No one, though, has ever asked the question quite as bluntly – or as specifically – as this. I try to stall. What should I say to her?

"I don't know," I reply, searching her face. There does not appear to be another question below the surface, and I can see she is not frightened. "I'm certain that the time is getting very close," I falter. "It might be today, but I'm not sure."

She smiles. "That's okay," she says. "I'm ready." Her

grip softens, and she closes her eyes. "God is good! I've had a wonderful life."

"My goodness," I reply. I relax now, as well. "Your life has been special in many, many ways." Within a few moments, she drifts back to sleep.

What, I wonder, *triggered her question?* She knows that my work with cancer patients has given me ample opportunity to accompany families as the end approached. Maybe she thinks I have some special insight, although my ability to predict the future is spotty. On the other hand, she has had plenty of experience with death. Over the past decade, her schedule has been packed with funerals and she has written dozens of sympathy cards. Her husband and nearly all of her friends are gone.

She does not, in fact, die that afternoon. The next evening, though, while the TV in her hospital room shows her Bears closing in on a Monday Night Football victory, her heart beats its last.

The rest of the world goes on, but for a time, my world stops. Memories of our lives together – times of joy and times of great challenge – sweep over me, and I find myself immersed in gratitude and sorrow. My family and I complete arrangements for my mother's funeral, a task made easier by her grace, her faith, and the simple gift she gave us when she looked at me and said, "I'm ready."

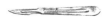

Point of View

Your most unhappy customers
are your greatest source of learning.
- Bill Gates

I hand out a short story to the fifteen residents and students. They follow along as one of them reads aloud:

> *"One last blow, and, blind as Samson, the black man undulates, rolling in a splayfooted circle. But he does not go down. The police are upon him then, pinning him, cuffing his wrists, kneeing him toward the van. Through the back window of the wagon – a netted panther."*

I am working to integrate narrative into medical education. During this early morning conference, the otolaryngology residents and a few medical students concentrate – heads down, brows furrowed – as they take turns reading aloud "Brute" by Richard Selzer, a riveting first-person fictional short story of an exhausted young surgeon who must repair the gash on a prisoner's forehead in the middle of the night. Both the surgeon's frustration and his admiration of the patient escalate as the roaringly drunk Black man "spits and curses and rolls his head." After one last, unheeded demand to "Hold still!" the surgeon calmly sews the man's ears to the cart, wipes the blood from the man's eyes, and grins victoriously down into his face, a demeaning gesture the surgeon profoundly regrets twenty-five years later.

The reading ends and everyone's eyes widen. The trainees are well on their way to becoming surgeons, and they squirmed as they read the story from the surgeon's point of view. "So," I ask the group, "what are your reactions?" After a pause, the discussion flows. Residents nod knowingly, recalling difficult, late night encounters with uncooperative, ungrateful people. "God," says a resident close to completing her five-year training, "those situations are really frustrating. I know exactly how he feels." Some of the students – having never been in the ER with a drunk person – wonder aloud, "But what do you actually do?" and, "Do you think this is a real story? Did this really happen?" I break off the discussion at the end of the hour. Several thank me as they file out. We have all been given something to contemplate.

A couple of days later, one of the senior residents, Tristan, and I are in the operating room. "Dr. Campbell," he says, "Melissa was upset by the story."

"Really?" Although Melissa is a junior resident, she should have already had similar encounters. "About the way the surgeon reacted?"

"Talk to her."

Later that day, I track her down. "Melissa," I ask, "do you want to talk?"

"Dr. Campbell." Her gaze is steady, and she speaks very evenly. "I was really disturbed when the writer portrayed the Black man as an animal. It was awful."

Oh, my goodness. Melissa is of mixed-race heritage. She is a gifted writer and a gentle soul.

"Tell me more."

"I hated how the writer described the victim. I was upset. I called my parents to talk about it, and they said I should talk to you. I wasn't going to. I didn't want to talk."

"Sorry," I reply. "Tristan ratted you out."

We spend time talking through the reading and her reaction. Where I had always viewed the story through the surgeon's eyes, she had immediately identified with the patient. "I apologize," I say. "I have always seen the victim's race as irrelevant to the arc of the story."

"Not me," she says.

As we talk, I remember that I have used the story "Brute" in teaching sessions before, but I cannot recall if other residents and students of color participated. If they did, were they upset, as well?

Without recognizing the harm, I have perpetuated a racist act of prejudice, a microaggression. *How often have I done this? Who have I hurt?* I see in a new way that, as a late-career, white male surgeon "authority figure" who grew up in a certain time and place, bringing my own preconceptions to every experience can spread as much harm as it can light. As I continue to work with residents and students, I will try to always remain open to what they teach me, as well.

"I'll find a different story next time," I tell her, "or maybe you can help me teach it in the future."

She smiles. "I'll think about that," she says as she checks her pager. "Excuse me, Dr. Campbell. I've gotta go to the ER. We'll talk more later."

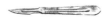

One After Another

It's in our interest to take care of others . . .
To help others takes courage and inner strength.
- Dalai Lama

I am working side by side with three Kenyan ENT doctors and a group of fellow Americans for our yearly ENT camp in Eldoret, Kenya. An elderly, emaciated man sits slumped in the ENT clinic exam chair. His eyes are sunken, and he winces whenever he tries to swallow.

"How long has he been like this?" I ask. "When did he start losing weight?"

The family members confer in Kiswahili. "He hasn't been able to eat for about six months. He has too much pain in his mouth."

I flip on my headlight and speak to his son who is fluent in both Kiswahili and English. "Please ask him to open up. I would like to look inside."

His son translates, and the man's mouth opens, revealing a deep crater where his tongue had once been. There is no movement of the remaining tissues. The ulcerating mass has grown into the lower jaw.

"We do not have a biopsy," I say, "but this is likely a very large cancer. It has been there for a long time." I run my fingers up and down his neck and can feel several enlarged lymph nodes on both sides lying just deep to the skin. "The cancer has spread to many of the lymph nodes, as well." Given the number of nodes involved, I realize that there is a strong probability that the cancer has already traveled throughout his body.

"In addition," says the son, "he is also HIV positive."

I turn to my colleague. "This is a very advanced cancer. Even without HIV, we would not have much to offer in the States."

"Really?" he asks me. "Couldn't you take out the cancer and rebuild his jaw and tongue with one of those big reconstructive flaps like you do in the States?"

I consider how best to answer his question. The kind of surgery he has mentioned takes a large team and ten or more hours of OR time. Recovery is prolonged and requires specialized nursing care and rehabilitation. The six weeks of daily radiation therapy treatment he would need after surgery is only available several hours away in either Nairobi or Kampala. He is emaciated and malnourished. I cannot imagine that he would be able to tolerate any sort of treatment, much less survive the surgery.

"No," I say. "In the States, we would probably arrange for a feeding tube, talk to the supportive care and infectious disease teams, and maybe think about some chemotherapy if he got a lot stronger."

"Does that help?" my Kenyan colleague asks.

"Well," I admit, "rarely. But you never know."

My Kenyan colleague turns to the family and speaks to them in Kiswahili for a couple of minutes. The elderly man nods, slowly rises from the exam chair, and walks back to the crowded hallway.

"What did you tell them?" I ask.

"We will arrange for a meeting with the palliative team. We will not try to treat his cancer."

I am surprised that there is a palliative team but, reflecting later, realize that Kenya and most of sub-Saharan Africa was devastated by HIV/AIDS just a few years ago. This medical center became adept at offering comfort when it could not offer treatment.

The exam chair is soon filled by another patient. And then another. Over the course of several hours, we examine adults and children with enormous cancers, huge thyroid goiters, and challenging problems. Many of them are scheduled for surgery in the upcoming days but some, like the elderly man with the tongue mass, are turned away because we have nothing to offer.

"Thank you for coming," I say to each of them.

"*Asante*, Doctor," they often reply. "Thank you. I feel better because you have seen me today," but I am the one who is healed.

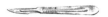

Horseshoes

*Those who suffer illness learn by hearing themselves
tell their stories, absorbing others' reactions,
and experiencing their stories being shared.*
- Arthur Frank

We stand together at the clinic room door, preparing to enter. The resident and medical student have already been in the room to meet the patient. "Tongue cancer. This is a seventy-eight-year-old man with an oral cavity mass and some memory loss. He had an ulcer on the side of his tongue for a few weeks which was biopsied at an outside clinic. No imaging yet. The lesion is tender. His wife died several years ago. He's in there with his daughters." The resident reviews what he found on the exam and runs through the list of potential treatment options. "Bottom line," the resident says, "I think he will need surgery."

I nod to him and begin to formulate my own plan in my head. Chelsea, the medical student, stands in our little circle of white coats. I look at her. "Any other details I should know about him?"

"Not really," Chelsea responds. "He's very quiet and lets his daughters answer for him. He is aware of his memory issues and seems to know that he has a problem. Except for the dementia, he's fairly healthy for seventy-eight."

"Okay," I say. "Let's go see." I knock and open the door. My new patient sits in the exam chair. His two daughters sit opposite to him. We all shake hands.

"I'm Dr. Campbell. You've already met Dr. Richardson and our student, Chelsea, right?"

"Yes, we have."

The resident sits down at the computer, ready to type his note. Chelsea finds an out-of-the-way spot in the very small exam room. Everyone leans in.

As in many situations when I am certain that getting to the bottom line will alleviate everyone's anxiety, I open with, "Let's jump to the end. So, from what Dr. Richardson has told me, you have a very early cancer. Stage I – the earliest we see. You will need surgery, but you have an excellent chance of being completely cured of this with surgery alone. Depending on what the pathologist tells us, you probably will not need radiation or chemotherapy."

The patient smiles weakly and looks at his girls, possibly seeking reassurance. "Surgery?" he repeats tentatively.

"That's good news, Dad!" His daughters are clearly happy to hear this.

This is where I usually review the medical history and then wash my hands to begin the examination. However, I need to know more about what he has heard and processed. I wonder how his personal story might interweave with his illness.

I sit before him and engage his eyes. "Where did you grow up? What did you do before retirement?" I ask him.

He tells me that he grew up a few blocks from where he

lives now. He never moved away. "I worked in a factory in my hometown. Before I retired, I worked in sales for a while." I note that he tells the story without enthusiasm. His voice is flat. His daughters confirm his story. *Well*, I think, *his long-term memory is intact.*

"Here's another question," I say. "What did you do for fun?"

Slowly, he raises his head and then a grin washes across his face. "Why," he exclaims, "I loved horseshoes!" He nods his head a few times. "You know horseshoes? I had eighteen ringers in a row one time! Can you imagine that? Thirteen another! You have to know how to throw the shoe!" Suddenly, he is standing up and bracing himself on the arm of the chair while letting his right arm swing free. With a gnarled hand, he demonstrates his technique in slow motion. "You grip the top of the shoe like this . . ." he pretends to be holding a horseshoe . . . "and bring your arm up like this. Here's the twist so that the shoe leaves your hand flat. It makes one rotation in the air before it reaches the stake." He whistles to let us know that his imaginary horseshoe is zeroing in on the target. "Then, PLONK! It drops down and you score! Then you do it over and over."

"That's amazing! Are you still competing?" I ask.

"Nah," he responds. "Not for a few years." The room goes silent, and he drops back into the chair.

"Dad, tell him about being in the state tournament."

"Oh, yeah!" He lights up again, describing some of his adventures. The worrisomely quiet man has become irrepressible. The key to him was horseshoes.

We finish the visit and arrange for his surgery. A discussion that might have been anxiety-provoking is easy and collaborative.

The daughters ask excellent questions, and the patient listens with a new level of attentiveness. He asks how soon we can operate. Soon, we are shaking hands again and they are on their way.

"What did you learn?" I ask Chelsea.

"That was really interesting," she says. "I know a lot more about managing tongue cancer."

"But," I ask, "do you know more about horseshoes?"

She laughs. "I sure do," she says. "That was amazing. He enjoyed telling his story."

And so, he did. Putting his cancer in the larger context of his life had driven the conversation. It took only a couple of questions for him to go from hesitant to animated; from being a man with a memory problem to being a former state-level athlete; from being identified as a tongue cancer to being a person with tongue cancer.

The conversation lifts me for the rest of the day. I feel renewed.

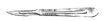

Gratitude

Life is a gift . . . every minute could have been an eternity of happiness! If only youth knew!
- Fyodor Dostoevsky

I'm sorry I had to break bad news to you today.

Thank you.

What for?

You guys gave me ten years. That's a lot of time.

But we haven't even started to treat your new cancer!

I know. But no matter what happens, I am grateful for the past ten years.

That's great, but we just took the cancer out back then. You did all the rest. But . . . um . . . what are you saying? Do you want us to treat the new cancer?

I suppose so. What choice do I have? I really don't wanna go through radiation again, but I'll do whatever you recommend. Oh jeez, that was rough.

Actually, radiation might, indeed, be part of your treatment, but the technology has improved a lot since the last time. They can focus the beam much more tightly than they could back then and spare most of the normal tissues.

Yeah, right. Easy for you to say, Doc. It's still gonna be rough, right?

No doubt.

Not surprised. No matter what happens, though, I'm still grateful.

Tell me more.

Before you treated me for my last cancer, I was a mess. I was drinking and smoking and living like there was no tomorrow. I got in trouble all the time. I was crazy. I'm amazed I was still alive. My family had given up on my ever being able to straighten out. I hadn't seen them in months.

I remember you had an attitude.

That's one way of putting it. Yeah, I came to those first couple of appointments drunk. I didn't know how else to face things.

So, what happened?

> I woke up the morning after you guys took out half of my
> tongue and realized that I had to change, or I was gonna
> die. It was that simple. Black and white. I realized I was
> gonna die.

But you knew that even making those changes didn't guarantee
that everything would turn out fine, right?

> I guess I knew it, but, at the time, I needed something to
> live for – my kids, my family, mostly. I was scared.

It worked out?

> Well, not completely, but for the most part, yeah. Losing
> part of my tongue was my wake-up call. Watching my kids
> grow up and getting to see my grandkids being born has
> been the best. I wouldn't have missed that for the world.

A lot of people do miss that.

> And that's why I say, 'Thank you,' even though you're
> sitting here telling me I have cancer again.

Well, then, I guess you're very welcome.

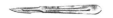

Gauze, Tape, and Love

He felt now that he was not simply close to her,
but that he did not know where he ended and she began.
- Leo Tolstoy

My patient and his wife are in my office for the very first time, and I can already tell that he will resist any display of sympathy from her, and she will clearly be uncomfortable with ever being a caregiver for him.

There is tension in the room. He "didn't listen" when she told him to get the spot on the inside of his cheek evaluated. She "went off and told the kids" without asking his permission. They speak over each other and past each other. Eventually, she looks at me. "We've been married forty-seven years, Doctor," she sighs. "We're both pretty set in our ways."

He grunts. After telling them that he will most likely need a feeding tube for a while after his upcoming surgery, they both make it clear that there is no way he will let her care for him and no way she will be able to do it. "Forget it," he says. "Why can't someone just come to our house and hook up the feedings three times each day?"

"I don't think the home care agency will do that," I say. "Many of my patients have worried about this. The nurses will teach you everything you need to know before you go home, and the home care team will make certain you are all set up in the house. The whole process is straightforward. You can both learn to take care of this very quickly."

She is adamant, as well. "Absolutely not! No way! What if some of the juices get on me? I can't stand it! Just the thought of having to deal with mucus makes me sick!" They glare at each other and then at me.

"Well," I say, "let's explore some alternatives."

They do explore several options, but soon learn that their choices boil down to either learning how to use the feeding tube or sending him to a nursing home for several weeks. They relent and resign themselves to working together. Arrangements are made, supplies delivered, schedules prepared, and jobs assigned. Life happens.

The surgery goes well, and he does, indeed, need a feeding tube while things heal up. After he goes home, I am surprised when they learn to adapt to the new routine. She becomes adept at taking care of the details of the feedings and then learns to help him through radiation therapy.

A few months later, unfortunately, the cancer returns in his cheek tissues. After an initial response to re-treatment, the cancer returns once again. Before long, there are no more curative cancer treatment options.

In addition to caring for the feeding tube, their routines now include weekly trips to the clinic and to the pharmacy. Caring for his facial wounds becomes a challenge. As his condition worsens, his strength wanes and his dependence on her grows. He is dying.

One day, they stop by the clinic for supplies. I ask how

things are going, and she answers most of the questions for him. She assures me that his pain is well controlled. He is weak but content. He is sleeping more and more.

He smiles at her. "I'm hanging in there, Doc."

I check the computer and see that the tube feedings are keeping his weight stable. I look in his mouth and measure the enlarging lymph nodes in his neck. A gauze pad has been carefully taped in place on his cheek, and I peek under the corner to examine the growing ulceration. The opening between his mouth and cheek skin – which started as a pinhole – is now the size of a dime. Saliva runs down his cheek. I replace the tape, but because the skin was wet, it does not stick very well.

After I finish the exam, I open the supply drawer and pull out some gauze and a roll of tape. I began aligning the dressing with the edge of the wound. The first piece of tape gives way as soon as I place the second piece.

"Here," she offers. "Let me take care of that."

I nod and step aside. She arranges the necessary supplies on the countertop and then methodically opens the gauze packets and snips pieces of tape to the proper length. He relaxes and raises his chin, presenting the gaping defect in his cheek to her. She cleans and dries the skin around the wound. After placing the gauze on his cheek, she guides his hand to where he can steady the dressing with his index finger, then adds one piece of tape after another to affix the dressing securely. Once she has inspected the periphery, she adds one final reinforcing strip of tape to the lower edge. The outcome is perfect. Not a piece of gauze has been wasted. Not a strip of tape is out of place.

She steps back and double-checks her handiwork. "There!" she announces.

He smiles again, then reaches up to assess the security of the dressing. "She's become quite a nurse, don't you think?"

"Indeed," I agree. "Very nice." My clumsy efforts to tape gauze to his face had been an attempt to dress a wound. She, on the other hand, was tending a relationship. Together, they celebrate how they care for one another using a ritual that involves gauze, tape, and love.

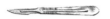

The Champ

I wasted time, and now doth time waste me.
- William Shakespeare, *Richard II*

Even though he was having trouble breathing and could barely swallow, he was too proud or stubborn to call either friends or family for help. Over the course of a few months, his weight dropped thirty pounds. His belt became far too long.

People had tried to help. His worried family members made several attempts to connect, but he always pushed them away with excuses for why they should not visit. "His voice started to sound so different on the phone! He wouldn't even open the door when I came by," the daughter told me later. Finally, after hearing one too many of his protests, she went to the house and pushed her way in. She was shocked by how he looked and by the condition of the house. She took him to a community hospital and, after a stop in the emergency room there, he was sent by ambulance to our medical center.

I meet him when he arrives. He is all skin and bones and is working hard to breathe. *Wow,* I think. *This man could walk through a harp.*

An examination and CT scan confirm that he has a very large, inoperable throat cancer. Because it threatens to completely obstruct his airway, we take him to the operating room for a tracheotomy and feeding tube. He spends the next few days in the hospital, getting accustomed to everything and recovering a bit. Plans for discharge are moving forward but, instead of heading back home, he will stay with his daughter. One of the sons is trying to get his house back in some semblance of order. The patient wants to be left alone and isn't very happy about the arrangements.

The day before discharge, I stop by his room and find him resting in bed. His children are talking, huddled in the corner. The scene is all too familiar: a concerned but estranged family with a lot of history, and a patient who has absolutely no interest in participating in his own care.

He coughs. They look over at him and sigh.

"Hello, everyone," I say. I glance at the bulletin board where the family has tacked up old photographs of the patient, his children, and his grandchildren. One photo in particular catches my eye. Five men stand in front of a bowling lane, hands on each other's shoulders and beaming at the camera in their identical shirts. The hairstyles, heavy-rimmed eyeglasses, and fading image confirm that the picture was taken many years ago.

"What's this?" I ask. "Tell me the story."

"Oh. That's from when Dad's bowling team competed in the national championships in Las Vegas." The daughter pulls the thumbtack and hands the photo to me. "He was one of their stars. If you ask him, he'll tell you that winning that tournament was the proudest moment of his life."

I hold up the picture and look back and forth between the photograph and my patient. Sure enough, one of the smiling, healthy men in the picture has the same eyes as the man lying in the bed across the room. Otherwise, he is unrecognizable. The bowling star's face is now gaunt, his biceps wasted, and the sleek black hair in the picture is now long, gray, and matted. His days of controlling the spin on a sixteen-pound ball appear to be behind him.

I notice that three of the five men have cigarettes packs in their shirt pockets. For me, the photo brings back memories of Saturday mornings spent at the bowling alley near where I grew up. I can still hear the balls rolling down the lane, the concussion as they found their pockets, and the rumble as they returned. I can conjure the odors of lane oil, popcorn, and cigarette smoke that permeated the entire building.

"That's amazing," I say. "I loved watching bowling growing up. National tournament? What an accomplishment!"

The patient beams. As he tries to say something, he begins to cough uncontrollably. When things subside, he signals his daughter for a pen.

He writes on his pad of paper in big block letters, then points at the photo and hands me the message. "WE WERE WINNERS." He shines a toothless grin and gives me a thumbs-up.

I tilt the notepad so his daughters can see what he has written. "That was a long time ago, Dad."

One of the girls shakes her head and points to photos of grandchildren and family gatherings. "He missed so much of this," she says. "Bowling, drinking, and being with his buddies was his life back then. A lot of missed opportunities."

He opens his eyes to look at her, wrinkles his forehead, and shrugs. I hand the notepad back to him, but he seems to think it best to not respond to her. He sets the pen back down and folds his hands. Soon, he closes his eyes and rolls to his side, facing away from his family. I return the photo to his daughter, and she tacks it back on the bulletin board with the photos of his smiling grandchildren.

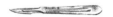

Waiting for Coronavirus

When you come out of the storm, you won't be the same person who walked in. That's what this storm's all about.
- Haruki Murakami

It is an afternoon very early in the COVID-19 pandemic, long before any vaccines will be available, long before any treatments have been approved, and at a time when case numbers are rising. The news is frightening, and no one knows what to expect. In the midst of this, one of my patients calls, and I know that I need to get him into the hospital *now*.

He has been recovering steadily from the throat cancer surgery I performed a month ago, until he started intermittently bleeding last week. The bleeding has continued – and worsened – since then. He drives in from out of town and shows me photos of what he has coughed up. It's bright red. *Arterial blood,* I think.

"There is a real possibility that this might suddenly become dangerous," I tell him. "We need to admit you to the hospital today. Now. We have to stop the bleeding before it gets worse. I don't want you to drive home."

"But, Doc," he replies, "what about the virus? I don't want to be in a place where there might be coronavirus! Isn't it more dangerous in the hospital than it would be at home? I had cancer, and I'm sure my immune system is weak. Isn't there another option?"

He and I have both been watching the news. Only a few cases of coronavirus have been reported in Wisconsin thus far, but things are really bad in New York and Seattle. The pandemic has overwhelmed countries like Spain and Italy in a matter of days. Experts warn that we are on the front end of a crisis. My patient wants to be as far from it as possible.

I had been reviewing my upcoming schedules with the office staff just before my patient arrived. We cancelled all of my elective surgeries to preserve gowns, masks, and gloves for our frontline colleagues. We moved routine clinic visits into the summer to prevent unnecessary viral exposure to patients and staff. We prepared for virtual visits to minimize the number of exposures. All of us are expecting the worst. My patient is right to be anxious.

"I hear your concern about the virus," I say to him, "but we'll do everything possible to protect you while you're here. I'll get you home as soon as possible."

I know he needs the bleeding controlled but cannot know with absolute certainty if the benefits of admission outweigh the risks of a possible infection while he is in the hospital. After more conversation, he relents and is soon on the way to a hospital room. I type up my note and head back to my office.

As I walk down the quiet, deserted hallway, I shudder, recognizing the same, unsettled churning in my gut I had during the early days of the HIV/AIDS epidemic decades ago. Back then, there was no reliable HIV testing, only a rudimentary understanding of disease transmission, and no effective treatment. AIDS cases were increasing rapidly, people were dying, and there was no end in sight. As a young trainee, I wore protective gowns and masks whenever I evaluated or tended to one of the shivering, emaciated AIDS victims. We read reports of health care workers at other hospitals contracting and dying of AIDS after puncture wounds.

One day in 1986, I plunged a needle deep into my thumb while operating on an HIV-positive patient. As the blood collected under my glove, I was terrified that I would be dead in a few months. I had a blood test to check my T-cell ratios. "It was a suture needle and not a hollow needle, so we don't think your risk is as high," the doctor told me. "Come back in four weeks, and we'll see if your counts drop." Until I was able to return for the repeat blood test, I feared I would leave behind my young family just as my career was supposed to be getting started. I was fortunate.

The memories that persist, though, are the sense of dread and the overwhelming uncertainty.

Scientists much smarter than me eventually elucidated the secrets of the SARS-CoV-2 virus and its variants, just as smart people eventually discerned the properties and treatments for the plague, cholera, influenza, polio, HIV, SARS, and Ebola after they first appeared. Each pandemic was deadly and left its mark. Before there was clarity about the disease or any available treatment, all that caregivers could do was be present, follow whatever guidelines were available, and hope that what they were doing was correct.

I am certain that caregivers accompanying the victims over the centuries each experienced gnawing uncertainty wondering, at some point, what was going to happen to their patients and, maybe, to themselves. Like my patient, they saw danger everywhere but did not know exactly what to expect.

My patient undergoes successful treatment of the blood vessel that had broken open into the surgical tissue. He does very well, has no more bleeding, and is soon ready for discharge. No fever, no complications, nothing bad. "Thanks, Doc," he says. "Really glad to be going home."

We bump elbows and he laughs. It's the new normal.

"Keep me posted," I say. I assume he will be fine now. But, of course, I don't know that with absolute certainty. Only the coming months and years will tell.

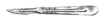

Determination

A tooth is much more to be prized than a diamond.

- Cervantes, *Don Quixote*

Adam possessed the look of a performance athlete slipping comfortably into middle age. He always greeted me with a hearty two-handed handshake. "I'm not giving up on this, Doc. It's just wrong. You'll back me, right?"

"Of course," I always responded, although we both knew he was facing an uphill battle.

He has always been very active – running outdoors or swimming most days – although the effects of the long-ago radiation therapy to his skull base for nasopharyngeal cancer ruined his balance and forced him away from the tennis courts.

He was grateful, though, to be a sixteen-year cancer survivor. To look at him, people would never have known that he had undergone a rigorous course of treatment in his early thirties. He had no external scars or marks. He was bright, energetic, clean-cut, and sharply dressed. Casual acquaintances saw a successful, handsome man who appeared in every way happy and healthy.

Until he smiled.

At every visit, we would talk about his battle to get his dental damage covered. "I was dumbfounded at the insurance company's response. When I had problems with my ear after the radiation, they covered the costs of the evaluation and treatment. When I had trouble swallowing, same thing. But with my teeth . . . that's been an entirely different story."

Adam's teeth were deteriorating, and his scrupulous regimen of brushing, flossing, and fluoride was unable to keep up with the decay. Flecks of enamel dislodged unexpectedly. Dental cleanings every three months were ineffective in holding the cavities in check. The dryness caused by the long-ago cancer treatment continued to inflict damage.

Adam's dentist submitted a proposal for ongoing care and extensive restorations, but the insurance company balked, sending his file to an outside reviewer, a dentist, for an opinion. That dentist reviewed the radiation reports, the photographs, the X-ray films, and the plan. "He said he didn't think my dental problems were a result of the cancer treatment! Maybe he's never seen what radiation can do to the mouth. In any case, based on his review, the company denied everything. They did offer to cover extracting all my teeth, but they won't pay for the extra care my teeth require now, and they certainly aren't going to pay to get them restored! I'm going to appeal. I can't go on like this."

Prior to his treatment, Adam never had dental problems, and now every tooth was ravaged. We reviewed a copy of the dentist's written report. "Doc, in your waiting room, I have talked to cancer patients whose teeth have fallen out after radiation. I don't want that to happen. I wouldn't be able to work with my clients anymore! These are my teeth! Why does my insurance company not consider my teeth to be part of my body?"

The answer sits at a major crossroad of US health insurance. When Medicare was enacted in 1965, the program specifically excluded several things that many elderly persons eventually need, including hearing aids, eyeglasses, and routine dental care. The Medicare statutes did make exceptions for any needed pre-radiation therapy extractions as well as for dental services needed while hospitalized. But routine care was specifically excluded.

Pretreatment dental optimization and posttreatment dental care after radiation prevent tooth loss and decrease the risk of osteoradionecrosis, a potentially devastating bone infection of the jaw. In 2000, the Institute of Medicine's Committee on Medicare Coverage Extension found that routine dental care for these post-radiation patients would save Medicare money in the long run by preventing complications and avoiding "the functional and quality of life problems associated with tooth loss." The recommendations were never implemented.

Private insurers followed Medicare's lead. Although Adam's coverage included medical expenses to manage other treatment complications, it specifically denied dental reimbursement except in cases of trauma and a few very tightly defined conditions. He learned that replacement can be expensive without insurance. For example, basic dentures cost upward of $1,600, and each implant adds at least $2,400. Many patients have no choice but to reluctantly go without.

This is not the first time that issues at the interface of the teeth and the body have vexed my patients. Many years ago, a realtor with excellent health insurance but no dental coverage refused to undergo general anesthesia for removal of a large benign salivary tumor because all of his incisors were loose.

"I'm not letting anyone stick one of those breathing tubes in my mouth," he told me. "I spend all day talking to people! If I lose my front teeth, I'll lose sales." Another patient whose oral cancer had arisen from the gingiva overlying her mandible had all her cancer treatment initially denied because a reviewer thought that her surgery and radiation therapy constituted "treatment of the teeth and gums." Another patient with facial contractures following extensive surgery and radiation required intravenous conscious sedation for any dental cleaning procedures. He struggled to convince his insurer to cover the extra services.

After a year of appeals, Adam's file was sent to the same reviewer. The request for coverage was again denied, this time with the comment, "It is difficult to say that the dental condition of all teeth is a result of the radiation treatment." Adam, with dogged persistence, worked his way up the chain, figuring out who made the determinations. He pursued additional appeals. He enlisted his caregivers to write letters and make calls.

Eventually, his file landed on the desk of someone familiar with the adverse effects of cancer treatment. The new reviewer agreed that the radiation had caused the dental deterioration and that the restoration of his teeth should be covered as a medical – not a dental – expense. Now, three years after the first phone calls and after a year of dental care, Adam finally has had implants, restorations, and crowns on all his teeth.

Dentistry and medicine diverged as professions more than a century before the 1960s-era decision that legislatively separated the teeth from the rest of the body. For Adam, the rift had practical and personal implications. Only by sheer force of will had he convinced his insurance company to cross that chasm.

"What a waste!" he tells me. "Persistence wore out resistance. It took dozens of letters, phone calls, and evaluations before they finally agreed to help me. Didn't that consume their time and resources, too?" He shakes his head. "I work for a life insurance company! I know the insurance industry and still had a difficult time getting this sorted out."

"Well, you won," I say. "Between the rules and the reviewers, other patients would have given up."

He nods. He understands that his remaining dental structures can still fall apart and that his dental saga is far from over. "I still worry about my teeth all the time. No matter what they say, my teeth are attached to the rest of me." He pauses. "But, you know, for the time being, I'm doing fine."

He grabs my hand in both of his, relaxes, and smiles.

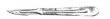

The Poor Historian

Historians are left forever chasing shadows,
painfully aware of their inability to ever
reconstruct a dead world in its completeness.
- Simon Schama

I notice that my new patient's wife and son are on the edge of their chairs as I start to interview him. He, on the other hand, seems distracted. "Tell me what you remember about how your cancer was treated," I say. "When did you have the surgery and radiation?"

"It wasn't a surgery," he tells me emphatically. "It was a biopsy."

"Harold, the doctor *said* it was a surgery!" corrects his wife.

"Yes, Dad. You have a long scar on your neck," adds his son. "That was an operation."

"No! They called it a biopsy, *not* a surgery! And it was two years ago."

"No, dear, it was five years ago."

"Five? Are you certain? That long ago? And I had radiation before the biopsy."

"No, Dad, you had the surgery first and then the radiation treatments. C'mon, don't you remember? You were still recovering from the radiation when the twins were born! And they just turned four."

"Are you certain?"

"Anyway, Doctor, he's been losing weight."

"No, I haven't!"

"Harold, your clothes are hanging off you!"

He scowls. "If you're so damn smart, then you answer all of the doctor's questions!" Things get worse.

Harold is the type of patient physicians tend to refer to as "poor historians." He can't remember his health history and has difficulty connecting the dots between his symptoms and his illnesses. His answers are unfocused, and he wanders off on tangents every time he begins to talk. It is hard to get people like Harold to complete health-related questions in a format that is easy to understand.

Dr. Jeffrey Tiemstra, in an essay entitled, "The Poor Historian," makes the point, though, that it is not the patient who is "the historian" – it is the doctor. *The historian sorts and organizes the past, identifying the important and meaningful events from the trivial, and then interprets the story in order to explain the circumstances of the present."* Tiemstra reminds physicians that it is their responsibility to make sense of the events told by the patient and create a record of the prior health history in order to safely develop a plan. Some days, the process of sorting things out and making sense of them is an enormous challenge.

Fortunately, Harold's outside hospital records are helpful. Later in the day, I will have more time to delve into his chart to reconstruct his cancer timeline to fill in the gaping holes in his memory.

For the moment, though, I lean back and listen to Harold interact with his wife and son. She is gentle but firm. His son is frustrated and tense. The way they talk to each other is another part of this family's narrative. I will need to know best how to share news, both good and bad, with them, and what I learn as I watch them in these moments will be helpful.

Some days more than others, I take my role as historian very seriously.

INTERLUDE

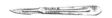

Boxes and Hyenas

My humanity is bound up in yours,
for we can only be human together.
- Desmond Tutu

Death is more palpable in this place.

We make rounds in the large, open wards of a district hospital in western Kenya. Beds often hold two people. The sheets are torn and thin. The room is warm despite the open windows; the flies come and go. Mosquito nets hang in tight balls above each bed, ready to be lowered at dusk.

We are *wazungu* – "people who wander aimlessly" in Kiswahili – and that is how the Africans refer to white people. Many Kenyans seem to believe that "the white doctors" are somehow better able to cure their illnesses, yet I know essentially nothing about the management of untreated malaria, tuberculosis, or HIV/AIDS, and everyone here seems to have one, two, or three of these diagnoses.

The patients look up as we pass. Some smile weakly. Some bow. Toddlers stare and reach. One man neither looks up nor moves.

The man's vacant eyes are unfocused. He is gaunt, yet his skin is taut – perhaps he is young. *He is dead*, I think, but no – wait –

he breathes, barely. The woman sitting on his bed follows us with her eyes but says nothing.

The nurses are friendly. They wave off our concerns about the lack of basic supplies. "These people are fortunate," they tell us, "because they or someone they know can afford the dollar per day charge for the bed or the cost of IVs and antibiotics." Most Kenyans never come at all.

As our vehicle leaves the hospital compound, I scan the businesses that line the road. Young men sit next to huge piles of shoes and t-shirts. Battered shipping containers have been converted into small shops and restaurants – called "hotels" here – but they all appear forbidding to a Westerner.

One of the small shops catches my eye. Two men are working out front, building some sort of rectangular furniture amid piles of planks and wood shavings. The piece appears to be a low table but, as I look more closely, I see that what I thought was a table is actually a handmade coffin. There are more ribbon-bedecked, freshly assembled boxes leaning against the shop's front wall awaiting people such as the young man we just saw up the road. Small boxes wait for the children nearing death in the pediatric ward. As we travel around the country, I notice other coffin stores, and they appear to cluster near hospitals. We notice many small cemeteries in the cities and rural zones through which we travel. They are all well-tended.

On safari, we are driven across the Maasai Mara – the vast expanse of grassland in Africa's Rift Valley that supports the giant migration of animals each year. Predator and prey, life and death, "The Circle of Life." "Animals die, and that is sad," we told our children back home when they were small, "but in death, life is sustained." They nodded in apparent understanding.

I ask our guide, who is not Maasai, about the people who live on the Mara. We have seen groupings of huts surrounded by makeshift stockade fences built to protect cattle at night from predators. Their nomadic lives revolve around the availability of water and forage for their cattle. They migrate to allow their herds to graze. "With no fixed homes," I ask, "what do they do with their dead?"

His eyes narrow, and he stares at me. "Did you see any cemeteries all the time we were out on safari? Did you?"

I try to recall. "No, I don't think so. No, I saw no cemeteries."

"The Maasai – they carry their dead outside of the compound at night and leave them in the bush for the scavengers." I catch my breath. "The ancestors of the Maasai," he tells me, "they are in the belly of the hyena." He lets that sink in. "The hyena," he repeats. Then he falls silent.

This is not the "Circle of Life" I shared with my children while we watched *The Lion King*. I spot another row of freshly assembled coffins back in town. They are brightly painted and decorated with fabric. They are beautiful and festive.

We return to our living quarters. The sky glows orange. Back at the district hospital, the lights are on but will soon flicker as the power fails yet again. A woman whispers, "*asante sana*" – thank you very much – as a nurse tucks the mosquito net neatly beneath her mattress and says, "Good night."

PART FOUR

Looking Back

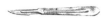

You are Here

"I don't want to get to the end of my life and find that I lived just the length of it. I want to have lived the width of it as well."
- Diane Ackerman

Nathan picks up a marker from the tray next to the dry erase boards. "Okay," he says. "Here's what he showed us."

The rest of our small group watches. Nathan is one of the more intense people I have ever met. He has been irrepressible during this small-group exercise for first-year medical students over the past few weeks. He has opinions on everything, some of which are a bit over-the-top, particularly regarding popular culture and the sports supremacy of his hometown baseball team. "Sometimes wrong but never in doubt," we might say about him.

Nathan takes the marker and walks down the length of the dry erase boards, creating a thick, black, fifteen-foot line from one end to the other. "Okay," he says again. "Here's what our college professor showed us. Now come up here and, each of you, take a marker."

We rise from our chairs and join him at the front of the room. "Now, which of you is the youngest?"

"I might be?" says one of the students, a shy woman who has gone directly from high school to college and then to medical school. She shares her birthday. Everyone acknowledges that she is, indeed, youngest.

"So, take the marker. Imagine that this line represents your life from birth to death. Left to right. Birth over there and death over here. Where are you on the line? Right now? What do you think?"

She blinks. "I dunno."

"Just guess. No wrong answers here. Draw a hash mark where you are."

She is twenty-two. "Um, here, I guess," she says, tentatively drawing a line about a quarter of the way across the board.

"Good," Nathan says. "Next?"

Everyone draws their own hash mark. One student worked for ten years as a systems engineer for a computer firm before applying to medical school. One spent six years as a middle school teacher. One earned a Master's in Public Health. Each one steps to the board and adds his or her hash mark to the line. "You, too, Doc." I am the oldest, by far. I take the marker and look at the line, adding my vertical slash a comfortable distance from the right-end terminus. I look at the hash marks and decide that the youngest figures she will make eighty. Judging by where I have added mine, I am hoping for ninety.

"Very interesting," Nathan says. "That's cool. But, think about this. What if your line is actually only this long?" He picks up the eraser and begins energetically rubbing out the thick timeline from right to left. Suddenly, my hash mark is at the far-right end of the horizontal line. He looks in my direction, shrugs, and keeps erasing, first to the engineer, then to the teacher, then to the MPH, and finally to the shy student right out of college. "Huh? How 'bout that? What if your line is only that long?"

He sets the eraser back in the tray and sits down. "None of us knows, do we? Any of us? Right? So, how do we react to that? As my professor erased the line, he kept saying over and over, 'How are you living today?'"

The room is quiet. As medical students and physicians, we submit ourselves to lifetimes of delayed gratification. We are forever looking to milestones: *How much longer until I finish training? How old will I be when I finally pay off my loans? When will I finally feel settled into a career? When would it be safe to start a family? What do I need to do to retire?* We're constantly looking to the next step. "Um, thanks, Nathan," I say. "Interesting exercise."

"Yeah," he grins. "*Carpe diem*, my friends. *Carpe diem*."

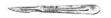

Degrees of Separation

The present time has one advantage
over every other - it is our own.
- Charles Caleb Colton

The cherubic young man smiles from the black-and-white class photo hanging in the medical school corridor. His open, relaxed appearance captures my attention. He sits on a wooden bench at the far-right end of the front row wearing a clean white shirt, a tightly cinched patterned tie, and a three-piece wool suit with stylishly wide lapels. He looks directly at the camera and could not be happier. Some of the other young men in the photograph have spontaneous expressions, as though they are reacting to a story or a joke. Two lean together mid-comment while a couple of others look away from the camera. I study the young men and try to imagine their lives.

I spend a few minutes searching for details. I surmise that the photo was taken in the afternoon because there are no shadows, and no one is squinting as they sit on the steps of the east-facing entrance. It is likely that they are taking a break from their studies and clinical work as they pose for their senior picture in front of the building where they have spent much of their past four years. As soon as the photographer releases them, many will likely run back up the stairs to the labs or lope down Wisconsin Avenue toward either Deaconess or Milwaukee Lutheran Hospital. For a moment in time, though, they are together as the camera captures the Marquette University School of Medicine Class of 1937.

I scan down the front row. Like four others nearby, the smiling student holds a cigarette between his fingers. None of the smokers seem to be trying to hide their habit from the camera. It will be twenty-seven years before the Surgeon General releases the report that definitively links smoking with cancer and seventy-two years before Marquette bans smoking from all of its buildings.

All the students appear to be white males. Most will end up in general practice, although an internet search tells me that a few will go on to other types of careers. I recognize a serious-looking student near the left end of the second row. He will serve in Guam during World War II and later be appointed the medical school's dean, eventually overseeing the transition of the school from Marquette to the Medical College of Wisconsin. Another will be an advocate for reforms in the automobile industry, publishing a futuristic article about safe cars in the June 1955 issue of *Popular Science* with illustrations of padded dashboards, collapsible steering columns, safety glass windshields, and instructions for how car owners can install their own safety belts.

The young man in the front row who has captured my attention is anonymous to me. He leans forward, robust and healthy. His career stretches out ahead of him; I imagine he sees nothing but unlimited opportunities. He won't think about retirement for decades. He and his sixty-seven colleagues, mostly in their mid-twenties, have finally arrived at the threshold of their medical practices, and they appear eager to get started. They are anchored in a different century, yet their smiles, anticipation, and camaraderie link them to all students of every era.

What does the young man think medicine will be like during his career? The first antibiotic, sulfanilamide, was introduced the year he was a first-year medical student, although it will be five years before penicillin becomes available and the word "antibiotic" enters common parlance. Medical innovations including radiation therapy, wound management, fracture repair, resuscitation techniques, and public health interventions are beginning to develop. He and his classmates are still recovering from the Great Depression, and it is safe to assume that each is aware of the worsening political climate in Europe.

These men represent medicine's equivalent of "The Greatest Generation." Social Security was only two years old when they graduated. Compared to my peers, the men in the photograph have very few well-studied drugs in their armamentaria. Deep understandings of genetics and immunology are years away. During their lifetimes, many fields including anesthesiology, oncology, and radiology will make enormous advances. Diagnostic testing in 1937 consisted mostly of a physical exam, plain X-rays, and basic blood, stool, and urine tests. Toward the ends of their careers, the economics of medicine will shift as Medicare is enacted and more than a few will likely lament the passing of "medicine as we knew it."

I do the math and discover that these vigorous, long-ago young physicians, if still alive, would be over a hundred years old now. Despite the distance and the decades, though, I also figure that many of them were reaching the end of their medical practices around the time I graduated from medical school in 1980. I do more math and realize that the Class of 1937 is as separated from me as I am from the young men and women in the Class of 2023.

My curiosity about the smiling young man with the cigarette sends me back to the internet. By comparing faces and hairlines in other class photos from online Marquette yearbooks, I think I know who he is. If I'm correct, he went on to marry, raise three children, and practice his entire career in Milwaukee. In 1954, *The Milwaukee Sentinel* reported that he bowled a 300 game. How closely did we come to overlapping? He died of heart disease at age sixty-eight in 1975, a month before I was accepted to medical school.

I exchange one last glance with the young man sitting happily on the steps, wishing him well with his career and his life. As I do so, a group of first-year students heads down the hallway toward the doors that will take them to the parking lot.

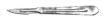

Discomfort

Put yourself behind my eyes and see me as I see myself.
- Rumi

Too many challenges, I think to myself. She lies on a bed in the trauma room, her eyes a bit too wide and her breathing a lot too noisy. Her grandma holds her hand.

"She was in a bad car wreck a few months ago," Grandma tells me.

My resident physician, Jenna, unravels the young woman's story. Nineteen years old. The wreck was a bad one; she broke several bones, suffered multiple injuries, and nearly ripped a large swath of skin off of her back. She was on a ventilator for a couple of weeks, eventually having a tracheotomy. After two months in the hospital, she went to a rehab facility. The tracheotomy was removed a couple of weeks ago, and the opening in her neck has almost closed up. She still has physical therapy and wound care every day.

"The facility says her breathing has gotten a lot worse over the past few days," Jenna tells me. "Here. Look at the photo."

Jenna shows me an image captured from a monitor when the young woman's voice box was examined. The vocal cords appear fine, but the space immediately below them in the top

of the tracheal breathing passage is nearly closed. Our young
patient has a severe obstruction of the airway right where her
tracheotomy tube had once been placed. If the passageway
closes any further, she will suffocate.

"Wow," I say. "We must get her into the operating room to
reopen her airway again. And soon."

This will not be easy, I think to myself. She is a very large girl
with a thick neck, and I am uncertain how easy it will be for her
to cooperate. Her scar is thick. I unfold the skin of her neck and
upper chest and look at the old tracheotomy site. *This won't be
easy*, I think again.

Soon, she is on the operating table. We are joined by our
intern. "Hello, David," I say.

"Hi, Dad," he responds.

My own son is one of our first-year residents. We have been
in the operating room together in the past, but I have yet to
figure out if I can balance the boundaries and responsibilities
of my roles as both parent and as faculty member. We spent
time together in the operating room when he was a student and
during a humanitarian trip to Kenya. Still, working with him at
my own hospital is a new experience for me. Especially on a case
where I am anxious about the airway and the outcome.

I know several other parent-child combinations in medicine
and have observed a few of them in action. Still, I am not certain
how having him in our residency program is supposed to work.
Will I *really* be able to think of him as I do the other residents?
Can I be objective as a teacher? Thankfully, I will never officially
assess his performance, but I will offer feedback to him as I
would to any other surgical trainee. As he develops as a surgeon,
I hope to view him as I do all of his peers, but I don't know.

The case begins. We will operate with her awake using local anesthetic because we don't think the anesthesiologist would be able to pass a breathing tube through the tight region. She makes a faint whistling sound, breathing noisily because of the tightness in her airway. Jenna numbs the neck, the neck is washed with a surgical soap, and off we go.

Jenna incises the skin of the old scar and we work our way through to the tissues below. "This is too thick," I say. "See how the cartilages are aligned? I don't see the usual landmarks."

We work carefully. At first, our patient is comfortable, but she begins to become anxious as we proceed. "Help me," she mouths, making no sound. The more we manipulate the cartilages of the trachea, the more anxious she becomes.

"More local!" Jenna numbs up more of her neck skin.

"We gotta get in the airway," I say. The dissection speeds. I direct my headlight into the enlarging wound. Nothing appears as it should. "The scar distorts things," I say. I put my finger in the wound, seeking a reassuring bulge of the airway but finding none. "Let's lengthen the incision."

We open things up more widely and continue. Jenna makes a cut where I direct, and a single rush of air escapes. "Good! There's the airway!"

No more air moves through the incision, though, and the patient's arms and shoulders start to thrash on the table. The monitor shows that the amount of oxygen in her blood is dropping.

"Here, David," says Jenna, "hold this retractor."

Holding retractors is the task that usually falls to the most junior person on any surgical team. A good retractor holder is highly prized. David proves up to the task.

I focus my light in the wound and finally spot some mucosa that looks like it should be the inside of the windpipe. Despite this, the patient is no more comfortable, and the oxygen level fails to improve. "We're going to have to try something different," I say. *But what?*

The patient is increasingly anxious. I worry that we will not be able to find an adequate opening. What if we cannot? We're in her trachea, but she is still unable to get air into her lungs! *What if we fail? What if she dies?* It could happen. *But my son!* I think. *My son is here. What if she dies while I am caring for her? And my son is here?*

And, with that, I experience my first moment when having my son in the program is somehow different than having any other resident. Losing a patient would be devastating enough, but I cannot fathom losing a patient on the table in front of my own son.

"We need to change tactics. See if you can get the rigid bronchoscope through," I say.

Jenna slips the scope in the wound and angles it toward the trachea. "I can't advance it, but I can see where it is tight!" she announces. "We're in the airway but still above the tight region."

That's why the patient isn't getting better, I think. The tight region is still below us. I peer into the wound but don't see the opening. "Pull up on the retractor, David." He does. And there it is.

"Give me a small endotracheal tube." The patient's chest is moving, but she is barely breathing.

The anesthesiology resident hands me the smallest tube she has on her cart. "Here's a 4.5."

David pulls up on the wound, Jenna concentrates the lights on the airway, and I force the tube through the tight zone. Air floods through the tube. The patient starts to breathe again. She stops struggling and relaxes. As do I.

With the airway under control, the anesthesia team is able to put the patient to sleep and we explore the wound, dilating the tight zone and getting a normal size tracheotomy tube back in her airway. A few minutes later, she is on the way to the intensive care unit with a secure, adequate airway. She has a long road ahead if she hopes to be permanently rid of the tube, but she has survived the first step.

She takes a deep breath, as do I. And my son is there to watch.

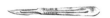

Our Local Medical Organization Disappears

All are needed by each one; nothing is fair or good alone.
- Ralph Waldo Emerson

I was an otolaryngology resident in the 1980s when a case of viral laryngitis left me incapable of speaking aloud. My mentor, a respected, senior member of our local Milwaukee Society of Head and Neck Medicine and Surgery, announced to the audience assembled in the University Club meeting room that, because of my incapacity, he would deliver my presentation for me. He gripped the podium and peered at the small crowd of friends, associates, and professional competitors. He knew them all well.

"Colleagues," he intoned, "before I begin, I must tell you something. I have been examining diseased vocal cords for almost three decades. I have seen all types of laryngeal pathology and disorders, acute and chronic, malignant and benign. Sadly, this resident . . ." he paused and swept his hand dramatically in my direction, ". . . this resident has the *worst* case of syphilitic laryngitis I have ever seen."

I was horrified but could not protest. Slowly, his lip curled into a half-smile and the meeting erupted in laughter. The presentation of my small research study lasted only a few minutes, but the good-natured ribbing continued for weeks.

During my residency, my fellow trainees and I looked forward to every gathering of the society. The meetings were informal, and it was our only opportunity to mingle with seasoned practitioners, connect names to faces, learn about their differing models of practice, and hear about their lives outside of medicine. I grew to admire the sophistication of many of the local nonacademic physicians. A few years later, as I returned from fellowship to start my academic practice, society meetings were where I nurtured professional friendships, talked about difficult patients, learned local history, and shared stories with people I might otherwise only have met over the phone.

At the time I had my bout of laryngitis, the society was flourishing. It had been established in 1975 in response to a malpractice crisis, and nearly every one of Milwaukee's twenty-five active otolaryngologists had joined and participated. The program committee invited speakers from state regulatory agencies, insurance companies, and law firms. Before long, the society began hosting nationally known medical speakers for well-attended dinner presentations several times each year. The typewritten minutes from the first two decades report strong participation and lively discussion. Each spring, there was a general interest meeting featuring a speaker, great food, and the participation of spouses. The spring meeting attracted such robust attendance that the executive committee sometimes worried if there would be enough space for everyone.

The society's most active era continued long after the malpractice concerns dissipated. An ever-growing cadre of community and academic practitioners met regularly to interact with visiting experts and to earn continuing medical education credits. Younger academic faculty built their local reputations and resumes by offering presentations and serving as officers. Residents attended for free, thanks to the members' generosity.

As time passed, the society's energy waned. The founding members retired, moved away, or died. Despite the growing number of active and retired otolaryngologists in the Milwaukee region (over eighty in 2021), membership and attendance dwindled. Scheduled meetings were cut from six to four each year, and the spring meeting – which at one time attracted seventy people – was cancelled in 2013 because so few people registered. Personal appeals to attend meetings went unheeded. In 2015, attendance fell to the point that the society's charter was retired and its funds disbursed. After forty years, The Milwaukee Society of Head and Neck Medicine and Surgery ceased to exist.

The society's experience parallels that of other groups both inside and outside of medicine. For example, North American memberships declined in service organizations such as Rotary International (down 29% between 2005 and 2014), Kiwanis International (down 28% between 2003 and 2015), and the Masons (down 31% between 2004 and 2016). Similar trends face churches, arts organizations, and social clubs. The loss has been attributed to a decline in "social capital," a term popularized by Robert Putnam to explain changes in society often brought on by shifts in technology and communication. In recent years, the American Medical Association's membership has continued to grow, but the large societies are likely vulnerable to the same pressures as the small.

It is difficult to know for certain why the organization failed, but several overlapping factors might account for its decline. Workforce demographics evolved over the years as the regional otolaryngology community shifted from solo to group practice and from general to subspecialty practice. The society found it increasingly burdensome to offer education credits, and there did not seem to be any viable alternatives to the traditional dinner meetings. Younger otolaryngologists were forced to decide between listening to an evening lecture or being present for school concerts, sporting events, or children's bedtimes. Older otolaryngologists believed they no longer had an obligation to or connection with a society that felt so unfamiliar.

A year after my poorly timed bout of laryngitis, I am able to present another small study, this time without mishap. After my talk, an older physician comes up and introduces himself. He is retired, after having been in a solo private practice for nearly forty years, and loves these local meetings where he can catch up with his old friends and colleagues. With a chuckle, he confides to me the unflattering nickname that my former chair earned during internship. Then he asks me, "What are your plans after residency?"

I pause. "I'm still deciding. I would love to do a fellowship in head and neck surgery and then come back here to be near family, but it doesn't sound like they will need me. I just don't know."

He smiles. "Is head and neck your passion?"

"Absolutely!" I respond.

"Then, by all means, pursue the fellowship," he says. "Everything will work out. Here's what I've learned: pick a career that brings you joy. You will wake up every morning, go to the office, and love what you do." He appears to sense my deep anxiety. "Don't worry," he adds. "There will always be enough work. Even if it takes time to get up to speed, your children will always have shoes. We are very fortunate people."

"Your children will always have shoes." That stuck with me. I took his advice, and he was right.

I understand that things must change, but I miss the camaraderie, the feel, and the experience of our local specialty society. It was an important part of my life as I was developing my identity as a physician. The Milwaukee Society of Head and Neck Medicine and Surgery was the place where I learned it was safe to lose my voice. And – as it turned out – the place where I found it, as well.

INTERLUDE

Rage Against the Answering Machine

How we spend our days is, of course, how we spend our lives.
-Annie Dillard

My grandchildren will never know the sound of a busy signal. It's true. The modern era has brought many miracles to our lives, including telephones that are always answered. When I get a busy signal these days, I redial, thinking there must have been some kind of temporary system overload problem.

Occasionally, a living human being answers my call. That is surprising, rare, and unexpected, though.

The third alternative is the most common.

I dial. After two rings, a prerecorded voice greets me. If I am standing, I sit. If I am sitting, I lean back. If I am leaning back, well, you get the picture.

"Hello, and thank you for calling Dr. Bob's office."

This phrase is fine. It's reassuring to know I reached the correct number. Whenever I visit Dr. Bob's office, I have a good experience. I really like Dr. Bob and his staff. Having the recording offer thanks for my call is courteous but not necessary. Knowing how kind Dr. Bob is, I find the message charming.

"Our regular business hours are 8:00 to 4:30, Monday through Friday."

This is useful information, but only if I had been calling Dr. Bob to find out when there is someone available to answer the phone. Perhaps having this information as part of the recorded message could help me orient myself someday if I suddenly awaken from a deep sleep not knowing if it is day or night. I'll call Dr. Bob's office to find out if it is daytime or not! If I hear the recording, it is probably dark outside. There are, of course, more efficient ways to determine this. I check my watch. It is 10:00 a.m. *Oh, no!* I think. *Why doesn't Dr. Bob answer? Is he hurt? Is everything all right?*

"If you are hearing this message during our normal business hours, it just means we can't get to the phone right now."

Thank God.

"Please be assured, we will take your call in the order in which it was received."

I like this phrase. An egalitarian approach to the seemingly trivial task of phone triage strikes me as a small moment of justice in an otherwise disordered, chaotic world. If someone extremely important called immediately after I did – the president, perhaps, or maybe one of the popes – I am delighted to know that Dr. Bob would take my call first. But I think to myself, *why do they take up precious time to tell me this? Is it really true? Might they be prescreening the incoming phone numbers?* Dr. Bob can see my name on the caller ID. He knows I am his patient. I half-expect a bored voice to click on the line and say, "Dr. Bob's office. We know who you are. Please hold," and then click off again. I make a note to check later to see if Dr. Bob spent the morning taking care of Beyoncé or Dua Lipa.

"Please stay on the line because our menu options have recently changed."

Now, I start getting restless. Is this message part of a nefarious plot to force me to sit in my chair for an extended period of time? Perhaps Dr. Bob is actually a front for a terrorist organization, and he uses these messages to get targets to remain in one place long enough for enemy snipers to train high-powered rifles on their victim. Why else would Dr. Bob try to force me to listen to the entire menu when I heard this exact same message two years ago? What's he up to? I creep along the wall and carefully close the blinds.

"If you know your party's extension, you can enter it at any time."

Why didn't they say this in the beginning? And why does Dr. Bob call people "parties"? When did "people" and "parties" become interchangeable? Is that proper usage of the term? Are there broader societal implications at play here?

"If this is a medical emergency, please hang up and dial 9-1-1."

I become alarmed. How stupid does Dr. Bob think I am? "Hey, Dr. Bob! I'm bleeding to death here!!! Got any quick advice??? Can you squeeze me in today and sew my arm back on??? Gawd, I hope you are taking these calls in the order they were received!!!" I am really starting to hate Dr. Bob.

"If you have a rotary phone, please stay on the line."

Rotary phone?!? Are they kidding? C'mon, Dr. Bob, who has a rotary phone anymore? Terrorists, perhaps? My kids have never even seen a rotary phone! And what if it's an emergency? Am I supposed to both hang up AND dial 9-1-1 on my rotary phone while my arm is hanging from its socket? While I'm bleeding to death???

"Otherwise leave a message after the tone, and we will get back to you at our earliest convenience . . ."

You will call me at YOUR earliest convenience?! That's probably true, but is it wise to TELL ME THAT?! I CAN'T STAND YOU, DOCTOR BOB!!!

Pause – Pause – Pause – Pause – Pause – BEEP

I grip the phone, grit my teeth, and record my message but suspect that the reason for my call has long since healed, ruptured, or metastasized.

I hang up, shaken and exhausted. Tomorrow, I will call Dr. Bob and see if he can help me understand why I am so stressed and no longer have time to get anything accomplished.

PART FIVE

Looking Forward

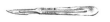

Recordings

*Knowledge is power. Information is power. The secreting or
hoarding of knowledge or information may be an act
of tyranny camouflaged as humility.*
- Robin Morgan

Not too many years in the future, I suspect, a patient returns home after a stay in the hospital. He powers up whatever device is the latest and greatest and clicks on "My Surgery."

"Let's see," he says. "I think I'll turn off the commentary for now. Maybe I'll watch it in HD and then try it in 3D." He scrolls to the point where his cart is rolled into the operating room. He blows up the image. Soon, he is toggling between images and videos recorded from several vantage points in the OR. The anesthesiologist slips in the breathing tube, the nurse tucks his arms at his sides with padding and a sheet, and the surgeon gets him positioned properly on the table. The nurse preps his surgical site. Once the skin is sterile, the resident places the drapes around the area. He clicks on the pause button as he watches the surgeon take a scalpel from the scrub tech. "Okay. Here we go!" The operation begins.

The patient splits the screen and calls up the anesthesiologist's monitor to see how his heart reacted to the surgery. He zooms in and watches his procedure from the first incision to the final suture, then runs the images in reverse to recheck the moment when the tumor was removed. *Whoa!* he thinks. *It was bigger than I thought!* On the screen, the resident balances the mass in her hand before handing it to the scrub tech. Finally, he lets the video run to the end when the team pulls off the drapes and he wakes up. He cringes. *Ugh*, he thinks, noticing how his face is flushed and creased. He speeds up the video images as he is slipped onto a cart and then rolled out the door and down the hall to the recovery room.

He switches to the recovery room nurse's perspective. *Jeez, I still look terrible*, he thinks just before watching himself throw up.

The cameras track him to the hospital floor and into his room. He studies the faces of his family members as they file in. He takes a few notes, amazed at how little he remembers of the entire day and the people he encountered.

He rewinds back to his surgery and turns on the enhanced audio. Closed captioning of every word spoken in the operating room scrolls along the bottom of the screen. The surgeon asks about everyone's weekend plans. The resident talks about an upcoming trip for fellowship interviews and her vacation. "I'm going someplace where my every move isn't recorded," she says, gesturing to the camera attached to her headlight.

"What the heck?" the patient exclaims. "Were they even paying attention during surgery?"

Though the technology is not fully in place, it would not take much to permit this scenario to occur. Video cameras are in every hospital operating room, ICU, and corridor. Many procedures are recorded. The only thing lacking is the software to fully mine and collate the data.

Digital technology has changed almost every aspect of medicine. When I started working in the 1970s, hospitals devoted large storerooms to paper charts and X-ray films. Every institution also had off-site storage for older materials because of the sheer volume of records. Retrieval of an exact file could take days and was often irrelevant by the time it was located. If something was misfiled, it was as good as lost.

A few years later, medical records departments began having old charts photographed, miniaturized, and stored on film before discarding the paper version. The technology certainly helped relieve storage issues by reducing large paper charts into a few sheets of film holding miniature photographs of its contents. Whenever I needed to review one of these old charts, I went down to the medical records department, requested the microfiche, and used one of the large readers to magnify the images. Unfortunately, many of the pages, usually including the precise page I needed to review, were so out of focus that they were impossible to read. I often thought that they might just as well have thrown the chart away.

In that era, the lack of reliably retrievable records often made it feel as though we were seeing every single patient for the very first time.

That is not the problem today. Although far from perfect, nearly everything is now digitally archived and available. Rather than keeping records locked away, patients can look up their own labs and reports. Endoscopic procedures, catheterizations, and arthroscopies are digitized. Information that once occupied long shelves of storage space lives in the cloud or fits on a thumb drive. Despite the communal gnashing of teeth by a generation of Luddite physicians like myself, the digital age has arrived.

In what ways might patients benefit if hospital workers knew that every action and word might be viewed by someone else? Studies in other industries demonstrate that workers comply with guidelines and protocols more often when they know they are being observed. Everyone washes their hands more often when they know that they are being watched. Despite the disdain for Big Brother, we would likely be more compliant with evidence-based protocols, more thoughtful in our patient care interactions, and more responsive to procedural coaching if we were accustomed to having retrievable recordings routinely used as a quality improvement tool. The simple act of observation improves outcomes.

Making recordings in hospitals is not new. Some hospitals have long employed photographers and videographers. Over the years, miniaturization and digital technology made the process simpler. In my practice, I capture digital videos of the voice box with a tiny chip camera on the tip of a flexible fiberoptic cable. Years ago, patients would come to the office with large cassette recorders, asking to record our conversations. These days, people record our visits on their cell phones.

In a twist on this approach, a Virginia man recorded what was said during his colonoscopy with his cell phone. According to an article in the *Washington Post* entitled, "Anesthesiologist Trashes Sedated Patient," he later discovered that the doctor had "mocked and insulted him as soon as he had drifted off to sleep," called him a "wimp" and a "retard," and had "placed a false diagnosis in his chart." The physician's behavior led to disciplinary action and a substantial malpractice settlement.

So, consider this: might we someday require every hospital worker to wear a body camera? What if every corner of the hospital had devices capable of capturing and archiving high-quality audio and the 360-video capabilities of an NFL football stadium? Once hospitals work through all of the privacy issues and regulatory issues, a host of individuals, including hospital administrators, lawyers, quality officers, and marketers, will find ready uses for the images and data they generate. Before long, patients will be reviewing their files.

This "open information" future represents the next phase of how our view of medical information will evolve. Physicians from the generations before mine believed it was ethical to hide dreaded diagnoses such as cancer and fatal infections from patients, but my peers and I entered the profession understanding that patients and their families are our partners in care and are entitled to more disclosure.

In the late 1980s, much of my work in the office was centered around teaching patients about their cancer. "Why do I have this?" "What are the options for treatment?" "What will happen?" "What kind of surgery will I need?" Sometime in the late 1990s, the availability of information – and thus my role – changed. As the internet age began and more people had access to mountains of health information (and disinformation), patients arrived at appointments after having first seen "Dr. Google." Office visits evolved from teaching people from scratch about their disease to explaining and disabusing them of what they had discovered online.

Increasingly, every bit of medical data – every report and

every note – is instantly available to patients. In a world of 24/7/365 video capabilities, physicians and nurses will no longer serve as data interpreters; much more data will be available to patients and families unfiltered and in real time. Artificial intelligence will provide analysis, and the health care workers of the next generation will likely be left pointing at screens and saying, "Well, there it is."

When policies mandating the immediate release of medical records went into effect, I began receiving more distraught calls from patients and family members, seeking reassurance or interpretation of pathology and radiology reports that I hadn't yet had the opportunity to review. To be very honest, I had trouble adjusting to this new world. I spent years being selective in what I shared from reports packed with coded medical jargon. Although I sought to be unfailingly honest and open, I believed that people could absorb only so much at one time and that knowing *everything* wasn't always helpful. I suspect the next generation will see that approach as reflecting a latent paternalism. In that sense, perhaps I am merely a younger version of the physicians of old whom I, myself, used to mock.

Our patient of the not-too-distant future settles into his chair and watches as the radiologist makes minor corrections in the computer-generated report from his scan. He watches, once again, the critical discussions held during his office visits and listens to the debates about his case at cancer conference. An algorithm samples the files and determines that the scan interpretation has a 93% chance of being accurate, the surgical duration was 17% longer than the median of similar procedures nationally, the recommended treatment was the same as would be offered at 83% of other medical centers, and he is eligible for seven different clinical trials at medical centers that are between 14 and 853 miles from his house. He jots down the information.

He clicks forward. After watching an ad, the screen tells him that, given his cancer stage, his other health problems, his insurance, his genetic profile, his zip code, his family history, and the treatment he should undergo, he has an 18.773% likelihood of still being alive in three years.

He sets down his pen, closes his eyes, and weeps.

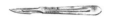

Artificial Intelligence

Medicine is a science of uncertainty and an art of probability.
- Sir William Osler

Two middle-aged men come to my clinic on the same day with symptoms of head and neck cancer.

Each reports several weeks of a slowly growing, painless, firm neck mass. When questioned, each has a very mild sore throat on the same side, but otherwise feels fine. Neither has ever smoked and is in excellent health. When they open their mouths, each has one slightly enlarged tonsil. Red flags are everywhere. Each has an absolutely classic presentation of an HPV-related oropharyngeal cancer.

Here are more things that they have in common . . .

Each sought help from a walk-in clinic near his home over two months ago. Each was placed on antibiotics and told, "You have a throat infection." Each had a throat culture (negative for strep) and was reassured that things should clear up soon but was also told, "You should call your primary doctor and set up an appointment if the sore throat persists for more than a couple of weeks." Each waited over a month beyond that because they thought the problem, based on the reaction at the walk-in clinic, was not serious.

In my practice as a head and neck cancer surgeon, these stories are frustratingly common. Because throat cancer is relatively rare, patients who develop symptoms are often thought to have more common problems. I have seen people with mouth and throat cancers arrive in my clinic months after their symptoms led them to have dental extractions, months of TMJ therapy, treatment for reflux, sinus medications, antiviral medications, and repeated courses of antibiotics. Ultimately, each patient experienced frustration, time away from work, unnecessary testing, and needless expense before coming to see our team. Because each person initially saw a different care provider, no one detected a pattern, but the scenario for each individual remained the same.

Of course, the people working at the walk-in clinics do the best they can. They have several patients to see and release over the course of an hour. Many people present with mild sore throats and swollen lymph nodes, and our mindset in medicine is that "common things occur commonly." Most people who pass through an urgent care clinic with a sore throat likely *do* have viral infections and not cancer. The doctors and nurse practitioners working in those settings would be wrong to send every patient with a swollen lymph node and mild symptoms for a CT scan and biopsy. They are correct to follow the adage, "When you hear hoof beats, think horses, not zebras."

But there are zebras out there. How might we help our primary care providers remain vigilant to unusual diagnoses? Or even think of them in the first place? How could we make our systems smarter?

Imagine this near-future scenario:

A young provider right out of training who has never seen someone with throat cancer encounters a new urgent care patient with a history and examination like one of the men described above. She enters the symptoms and examination findings into the electronic medical record system using a drop-down graphical user interface. The computer creates this summary:

> *This is a fifty-two-year-old otherwise healthy, non-smoking man with no travel or exposure history and two months of a slowly enlarging, painless, firm mobile 4.5 cm (1.8 in) right upper neck lymph node and mild right-sided sore throat.*

While she is considering which antibiotic to order, the system's database is searching through millions of patient stories and hundreds of thousands of peer-reviewed guidelines and journal articles. Her computer prompts her to ask a few questions she had not considered. For example:

> *Please ask the patient whether he has:*
> *Dental problems*
> *Difficulty with articulation*
> *Bleeding*
> *Ear pain*
> *Change in voice or articulation*
> *Change in swallowing*

The doctor completes the question prompts and hits ENTER. A screen pops up:

*Based on the constellation of findings, this patient has
an 81.4% probability of a Stage II or higher HPV-
related squamous carcinoma of the right oropharynx
(either tonsil or tongue base).*

The system then cross-checks the patient's insurance coverage
and home address, schedules an urgent CT scan, initiates the
authorization process, and offers a next-day consultation with a
nearby cancer team. It tentatively reserves a time for an ultrasound-
guided needle biopsy of the neck mass. If the provider has ordered
unneeded tests or medications, the computer politely suggests
that there are less expensive and more effective approaches. Before
the patient goes home, the system provides helpful, culturally and
education-level appropriate teaching materials, maps, and contact
information. The next morning, the system generates calls and
follow-up text messages to check on the patient and makes certain
that he keeps his appointments.

I suspect that we are not far from being able to accomplish
this.

Systems like this would have helped me be a better doctor. I
recall a patient who was eventually found to have throat cancer
but presented with such unusual symptoms that I was initially
drawn to think she had a non-malignant diagnosis. What if a
decision algorithm had been able to search through thousands
of patient scenarios and find a few others who had presented the
same way? Might I have immediately broadened my approach,
thereby shortening the time until I was able to make the correct
diagnosis?

Medical Oncologist Siddhartha Mukherjee, in a *New
Yorker* essay entitled "The Algorithm Will See You Now,"

envisions a future where we focus big data on clinical problems. As examples, he describes "deep learning" programs that assist radiologists and dermatologists to make accurate diagnoses. For example, machine-learning systems with thousands of images of skin lesions pick out melanomas more precisely than human dermatologists do. These types of algorithm-based systems might augment (or even replace) human decision-making in many specialties.

There are immense hurdles to overcome, including privacy and security concerns, data quality, and data throughput. Nevertheless, the potential to save money, resources, time, and – most importantly – lives, is real.

The mythical, kindly, old-school, independent general practitioner who relied solely on his (usually his) intuition and anecdotal experience was fading from the scene even when I was in training. Young physicians will soon barely remember paper-based books, journals, and medical charts. Each generation will have more powerful digital tools at its fingertips.

So, will we need doctors at all? Dr. Mukherjee shares a story of a dermatologist he followed during her busy day in the clinic. He notes that almost all her patients felt better after their appointments. "They had been touched and scrutinized . . . A conversation took place." The dermatologist does more, of course, than make diagnoses. "[She] spent the bulk of her time investigating causes. Why had the symptoms appeared? Was it stress? A new shampoo? . . . Why now?" Perhaps future generations of caregivers will focus less on making diagnoses and more on addressing the *why* of illnesses and the importance of remaining present for patients at critical moments.

Providing a diagnosis is not of much use unless we share what it means, what comes next, and the promise to share the journey. A computer algorithm might fulfill those goals someday, but I suspect that it will be a long, long time before it can.

The two cancer patients who came that day in my clinic did well. I continue to see them and talk about treatment side effects, but we also discuss their lives and families. I reassure them that things look fine, shake their hands, and stay available to them if they are ever concerned or scared. Let's see a computer algorithm do that.

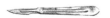

If Surgery Becomes a Spectator Sport

*"What's the worst thing that can happen to a quarterback?
He loses his confidence."*

- Terry Bradshaw

Wayne: Hello again, everybody, and welcome to our live play-by-play coverage of surgery! Today, we will watch two old adversaries battle it out under the bright lights within the storied confines of Operating Room 37. Larry, this promises to be quite a battle. What are you looking for in this matchup?

Larry: To be honest, Wayne, not much has changed since these two rivals last met. The surgical team – led by the twenty-year veteran surgeon – will take on the growing tumor. Overall, the surgeon seems to be holding up pretty well, but he has become increasingly intimidated by the technological bells and whistles that have entered the game over the years. I'm certain that he also feels pressure from the younger surgeons on the sidelines. Fortunately, the team has great depth at several key positions here in the operating room, and they are usually able to cover for his weaknesses. Wayne, I know that you think it's about time to bring up one of the rookies, but the surgeon still has some pro-quality moments. I agree with you, though, that he's not quite what he was in his prime!

Wayne: Larry, we'll watch closely and see how he does today. We've commented that he's been getting more flustered lately when things don't go perfectly. His future as a starter might be riding on what happens today. I was checking the scans just before airtime, and the tumor seems up to the task today. It is a real up-and-comer – full of surprises – and could prove to be a real competitor. It certainly has been displaying confidence and plenty of attitude. Final preparations are almost complete, so we will take a quick preoperative time-out. Thanks for joining us for the Pre-op Show! While everyone stands for the Time-Out Checklist, we'll take a quick break. Back in a moment for the big event right after this word from America's favorite beer. This is the Surgical Radio Network!

Wayne: Welcome back, everybody! We're ready . . . there's the incision! The surgeon makes a nice move, lifting the skin flap neatly and securing an extra hemostat in his palm. Outstanding work identifying the proper incision depth and managing all of the small vessels along the way! Perfect bipolar setting, I might add. Let's watch that again in reverse-angle slow motion . . . great exposure and every corner of the field is completely under control! Retractors are all at the correct angles, exposure adequate! Terrific tissue plane separation. As in each of these matchups, the first several moves are scripted. It looks like the team's strategy today will be to circle the tumor, rather than going right at it.

Larry: You know, Wayne, I like this approach. See how the surgeon squares up to the table and works from a balanced stance? Classic footwork. It's fun to watch an old pro go at it. He gradually brings in his newest assistant, giving her small responsibilities and plenty of positive reinforcement. Notice how he keeps his eyes focused on the field even as he tracks all of the activities in the room? Those skills take years to develop. He's off to a good start.

Wayne: Right you are, Larry! A big vessel just came into view, and he's moving confidently to control it. Slick dissection then "clamp, clamp, cut, tie, tie!" Perfect! That's another $500 for "Arteries for Charity" from our lead sponsor, America's Blood Banks! Back in a minute!

Wayne: We're ready to go again. Uh, oh. Look at that, though, Larry! Really poor technique there – far too much wasted movement. The lights are all wrong. His elbows are too high, and the resident's hand is blocking his line of sight to the target. It's all about maintaining discipline and control. Remember what happened last month during that thyroidectomy? He totally lost it after absentmindedly scratching his nose and getting a facemask penalty! Look how the student is being expected to retract when she can't even see the field. The surgeon must arrange his assistants more effectively in that situation. Whoa! Unbelievably, the surgeon just yelled at the scrub tech and threw a hemostat on the floor! There's a flag! He's claiming that the hemostat merely slipped, but the replay clearly shows that his arm was moving forward when the instrument left his hand. Despite his experience, his head is not in the game right now. Very poorly played.

Larry: I agree, Wayne. Wisely, he's calling for another time-out to let things settle down before he stumbles yet again. Reset the retractors; turn down the music.

Wayne: There's plenty of time to get things under control. While the last play is under review, we'll take a break. Back in a moment after a word from America's favorite line of full-size pickup trucks.

Wayne: We are deep into the second half now. Things have turned around, and the resident has really stepped up her game. You can sense that the surgeon and resident are in complete sync now. Several great moves with barely a word spoken between them. Whoa! Oh, my goodness, Larry! Suddenly there is blood all over the field again!

Larry: He must remain calm! Wayne, you can sense how tired he is. He's reaching for more sponges! Direct pressure. This looks dicey.

Wayne: I agree, Larry. We are four hours into this thing, and the tumor is roaring back! The momentum has shifted, and it is time to discard the textbook. He has to step up and innovate. It is all about defense now. The team must concentrate on bringing consistent pressure and looking for opportunities to turn things around.

Larry: Y'know, Wayne, that move by the tumor was *completely* predictable. The surgical exposure remains suboptimal, and his technique is getting sloppy. Other teams would have deployed the Lone Stars long ago or brought in another set of hands on the Army-Navys. Small steps are needed. This is a grind-it-out, short-yardage situation. He needs to go back to the basics. Look at the surgeon: his posture has deteriorated. Clearly, fatigue is becoming an issue. Not a pretty picture. There's an official time-out for a blood loss measurement.

Wayne: Well, Larry, we'll take a quick time-out, as well. Back in ten seconds after station identification. This is the Surgical Radio Network.

Wayne: We're back again. Limping toward the final moments now! Yes! The tumor is completely separated from its blood supply! The last cuts are complete! THERE IS YOUR SCALPEL! It's all over but the closing music!

Wayne: Whoa-boy! The surgical team defeated the tumor but I gotta tell you, Larry, this was a nail-biter right up until the end. My sense is that they will have to rethink their entire approach before the next case – this one could have gone either way. Not the surgeon's greatest performance, don't you agree?

Larry: I'm totally with you, Wayne. There will be hard questions about several of the decisions he made today. I mean, they got the desired outcome, but – c'mon! – it wasn't pretty. The commentators will be brutal tomorrow.

Wayne: Right you are, Larry! So, that's it from Operating Room 37. Stay tuned! Following some updates from the other ORs, we'll be back in a few minutes for our Post-Op Show with interviews from the locker room. We will also take a first look at the crop of young surgeons coming out of fellowships and check our experts' predictions on the upcoming draft. Thanks again for joining us for this live broadcast! Until next time, this is the Surgical Radio Network.

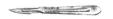

Suture Removal in the Mid-Twenty-First Century

The future of robotic surgery can be determined only by probing the possibilities. To ignore the potential for extending the boundaries and safety of surgical care with robotic technology seems unwise.

- Bulletin of the American College of Surgeons, 7/2013

It is a spring morning in July 2047. Dr. Aiden Smith enters the clinic room and greets Rebekah, the nurse, who is sitting at the room's control panel. "Good morning, Rebekah! Remind me who our first patient is? What did she have done?"

"Good morning, Doctor. This is Mrs. Morgan. You performed a thyroidectomy on her last week."

Mrs. Morgan opens her mouth to say something, but Dr. Smith doesn't notice. "Well, let's take a look at the incision." He turns to Rebekah and speaks under his breath. "We performed this robotic surgery through her belly button."

Rebekah helps Mrs. Morgan lie back and exposes the incision. Dr. Smith dons a headset with the words "Clinic Room Operational Computerized Upload Synthesizer" emblazoned on the side. He speaks into the headset. "CROCUS, create a microscope."

A wall panel opens, and a 3D printer appears. Within seconds, a fully functional operating microscope custom fitted to Dr. Smith's inter-pupillary distance and left-handedness emerges from the printer. A robotic arm grasps the microscope and brings it to eye level. Dr. Smith looks through the eyepieces and examines the umbilical wound carefully.

He begins to dictate his report. "Everything is healing well. The incision is clean and dry. Both stitches are intact. No evidence of any postoperative complications."

Mrs. Morgan is startled when a computerized voice announces, "The patient's insurance coverage allows for one post-thyroidectomy fiberoptic laryngeal examination to assess vocal fold movement and function."

"I almost forgot," Dr. Smith mumbles. He adjusts the controls and speaks into the headset. "CROCUS, deploy the laryngoscope."

The examination table creates a vacuum between itself and Mrs. Morgan that prevents her from moving. A nano-camera on a fiber emerges from the microscope and slips into her right nostril, advancing quickly into her throat. Dr. Smith looks at the images on the screen. "Both vocal cords are mobile," he says. "Umm . . . there is a brisk gag reflex."

"CROCUS, remove the microscope." The nano-camera retracts, and the robotic arm drops the microscope down a chute in the wall. A whooshing sound is heard. The billing total updates.

Rebekah taps Dr. Smith on the shoulder. "Why did you close her incision with stitches? I haven't seen you use suture since I started working with you! You usually use a bioengineered, genetically-compatible adhesive."

"Glad you asked, Rebekah! The rep told me about a new suture removal technique, and I wanted to try it out. Watch this!" He speaks into the headset. "CROCUS, create a Robotic Suture Removal Device."

The 3D printer begins working furiously. A robotic control panel emerges. Dr. Smith sits down at the console and looks through the eyepieces, his back to Mrs. Morgan. Next, a full-size surgical robot emerges. The arm yanks it over the exam table. As it does so, a puff of smoke emerges from the side of the robot. Mrs. Morgan frowns as she watches wisps of smoke continue to appear.

"See, Rebekah? In the past, I sometimes pulled too hard when I removed sutures by hand. The company claims that this approach is more precise, causes less pain, and improves patient satisfaction survey results."

Two robotic arms emerge, one with a diamond-tipped micro-dissecting scissor and the other with a laser-cut articulated precision-matched jeweler's forceps. The billing total updates. The robot grasps the first stitch and cuts the suture just below the knot. The billing total updates again.

Mrs. Morgan, who has been watching smoke pour steadily from the robot, now notices sparks. She passes out. The robot is quickly engulfed in flames. The sprinkler system activates. Everyone is drenched.

"Dr. Smith!" Rebekah shouts over the deluge. "Mrs. Morgan has fainted! Move the robot so I can get to her!"

Dr. Smith turns with surprise. "CROCUS, extinguish and discard the robot."

Alarms sound and strobes flash. The flaming robot, now engulfed in steam, disappears down the chute. A whooshing sound is heard. The billing total updates.

"Wow, Dr. Smith, that was close! But she still has one stitch left."

"Well, let's move her to another examination room and print another robot. I don't think it would be safe in here with three inches of standing water."

"Good thinking, Dr. Smith. Safety first! By the way, you failed to initiate the Time-Out Checklist before the suture removal."

Dr. Smith looks at her in horror. "Oh, no! I forgot to initiate a Time-Out? Not again! That's the third time this year!"

The 3D printer springs to life, and the robotic arm grabs Dr. Smith, holding him in place as it prints a jail cell which quickly encases him. He sits helplessly on the hard bench, pulls the rough wool blanket around his shoulders, and drops his head into his hands. "Now I'll never get my charts finished!"

The power supply for the examination table shorts out, which releases Mrs. Morgan. As Rebekah contemplates Dr. Smith's fate, Mrs. Morgan carefully steps down from the table and quietly sloshes out the door.

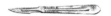

To Know When It's Time

Incompetence is the true crisis.
- Albert Einstein

Some patients find reassurance in gray hair, or so it seems.

As a sandy-haired, junior faculty member in my mid-thirties, I make rounds with one of our resident physicians. Although he is still in his late twenties, he has a full head of very prematurely gray hair. We stop in to see an older patient to "staff" the case – that is, have the resident present the patient's story to me as the faculty physician. We enter the room and introduce ourselves. "Mr. Smith," the resident says, "This is Dr. Campbell. He is my professor."

The man looks back and forth between the gray-haired resident and me.

"Yeah, right!" the patient says. "You're a professor. Sure. Who is he, really?" At the time, the TV show, *Doogie Howser, MD*, is still on the air. More than once, I have been told that I look a bit like the sixteen-year-old titular character. Despite my reassurances, the patient remains skeptical.

I knew, of course, that my days of looking too young to be a doctor were numbered. I don't remember when I last heard the comment, but it has been decades since anyone was confused about whether I have enough years behind me to do what I do.

Now, I think more about the other end of the career. When is a physician too old to continue?

An article in the *Annals of Surgery*, entitled "The Aging Surgeon," helped bring the topic into better focus for me. The authors recounted the story of Dr. Ferdinand Sauerbruch, an inventor of medical devices and a giant of surgical innovation. He began his career after graduating medical school in 1902, developing innovative limb prostheses for World War I soldiers and creating a pressure chamber that advanced the practice of thoracic surgery. He served as chair of surgery at Berlin's Charité Hospital from 1927 to 1949 and frequently cared for the rich and famous because of his technical prowess. He knew Hitler and, although he is credited with supporting victims of persecution and opposing the "euthanasia programs," his relationship to the Nazis has been referred to as "ambiguous."

Dr. Sauerbruch is also known for his horrific decline. In 1948, toward the end of his career, he began showing signs of dementia; in the operating room, he was noted to be erratic, forgetful, moody, and technically inept. He caused immeasurable harm during even simple procedures. Despite being encouraged to do so, he refused to retire. Unfortunately, his iconic stature apparently allowed him to keep operating in his hospital until a famous actor died during a procedure. He was prevented from working in the hospital but continued to perform surgery in an OR he built in his home until he died in 1951.

Surgeons are subject to the same aging issues as everyone else. We all experience declining sensory functions, a loss of habitual and controlled analytic memory, and decreased visual-spatial abilities. Despite this, many surgeons, when asked, do not believe that they are in decline. As Dr. Sauerbruch's story confirms, declining function and an absence of insight is a dangerous combination in a surgeon when other people's lives are at stake. There is enormous variability between individuals, but this decline is the basis for mandatory retirement at age sixty-five for commercial airline pilots, fifty-seven for FBI agents, and fifty-five for air traffic controllers. There are, interestingly, no such age-based retirement requirements for American physicians.

During my early years working as a nursing assistant in our local hospital, I observed some of the older doctors, many of whom had been on staff for decades. At the time, we viewed the oldest of the physicians as either cantankerous, doddering, or harmless. The older surgeons tended to be in the cantankerous category. In retrospect, we gave them labels for good reason.

A few years later, my fellow trainees and I christened the various surgeons under whom we trained as cranky, wise, rigid, steady, inscrutable, or timid. Some of the older doctors "still had it," and others did not. Doing the calculations now, I realize that many of them were younger then than I am now, even as I continue to work and perform surgery.

I experience a twinge every time I can't recall a person's name or it takes longer than it should to recall where I left a notebook. I look in the mirror and see only gray. I understand that this wonderful opportunity to perform and teach surgery will not, and should not, last forever.

Surgeons hear a lot of great things about themselves from patients and family members. I know that my coworkers tend to be positive or keep quiet. Now that I have read about Dr. Sauerbruch, I am more committed than ever to step aside while I am still safe. I only hope that when someone sees that I am not providing the absolute best care possible, my friends and colleagues will tell me.

And that I will believe them.

Notes

Commencement

Newton BW, Barber L, Clardy J, Cleveland E, O'Sullivan P, Is There Hardening of the Heart During Medical School? *Academic Medicine* 2008 (Mar);83(3):244-249. https://journals.lww.com/academicmedicine/Fulltext/2008/03000/Is_There_Hardening_of_the_Heart_During_Medical.6.aspx

Mistakes

To Err is Human: Building a Safer Health System, Institute of Medicine Committee on Quality of Health Care in America; Editors: Linda T. Kohn, Janet M. Corrigan, and Molla S. Donaldson. Washington (DC): 2000. https://pubmed.ncbi.nlm.nih.gov/25077248/

The Phone Call

Excerpt from "Grief" by Barbara Crooker. From the Poetry Foundation. https://www.poetryfoundation.org/poems/88766/grief-56e86db5ba0be

Across the Divide

Wendell Berry, Health is Membership. http://tipiglen.co.uk/berryhealth.html

To Enable Well-Being

Atul Gawande, *Being Mortal: Medicine and What Matters in the End*. Metropolitan Books, Henry Holt and Company, New York: 2014. http://atulgawande.com/book/being-mortal/

Point of View

Selzer R, Brute. *The Doctor Stories*. Picador, New York 1999.

The Book

Robert Coles (in the introduction to) William Carlos Williams, *The Doctor Stories*. New Directions Press, 1984.

Determination

Center for Medicare Advocacy. *The Medicare Dental Exclusion: Is It Being Used to Deny Vulnerable Beneficiaries Needed Care?* Published online May 2015.

Medically necessary dental services. In: Field MJ, Lawrence RL, Zwaniziger L, eds. *Extending Medicare Coverage for Preventive and Other Services*. Institute of Medicine, Division of Health Care Services, Committee on Medicare Coverage Extensions. Washington, DC: National Academy Press; 2000. https://www.ncbi.nlm.nih.gov/books/NBK225259/

The Poor Historian

Tiemstra, J, The Poor Historian, *Academic Medicine* 2009 Jun;84(6):723. https://journals.lww.com/academicmedicine/fulltext/2009/06000/the_poor_historian.18.aspx

Waiting in Line
  Paul Farmer, *Pathologies of Power*. University of California
  Press, 2003.

Our Local Medical Organization Disappears
  Rotary International Regional Membership Supplement.
  USA Canada Caribbean Islands 2013 https://my.rotary.
  org/en/document/regional-membership-supplement-
  USA-Canada-Caribbean-Islands. Accessed September 10,
  2018.

  Erickson J, Broderick B. Kiwanis International Dues
  Increase. PowerPoint Presentation to the 2015 Kiwanis
  International Convention: http://www2.kiwanis.org/docs/
  default-source/conventions-events/KI-2015/downloads/
  icon_duesincrease_2015-pdf.pdf?sfvrsn=2. Accessed
  September 10, 2018.

  Masonic Services Association of North America. Masonic
  Membership Statistics 2015-2016. http://www.msana.
  com/msastats.asp. Accessed September 10, 2018.

  Robert Putnum, *Bowling Alone: The Collapse and Revival
  of American Community*. Touchstone Books, Simon &
  Schuster. 2001

Recordings
  Anesthesiologist trashes sedated patient, *Washington Post*,
  June 23, 2015 https://www.washingtonpost.com/local/
  anesthesiologist-trashes-sedated-patient-jury-orders-her-

to-pay-500000/2015/06/23/cae05c00-18f3-11e5-ab92-c75ae6ab94b5_story.html

Artificial Intelligence
Siddhartha Mukherjee, The Algorithm will See You Now, *New Yorker*, May 2017. https://www.newyorker.com/magazine/2017/04/03/ai-versus-md

To Know When It's Time
Katlic MR, Coleman J, The Aging Surgeon, *Annals of Surgery* (Aug) 2014; 260(2): 199-201 https://journals.lww.com/annalsofsurgery/Fulltext/2014/08000/The_Aging_Surgeon.1.aspx

Prior Publication

Previous versions of some of the essays in this collection have appeared elsewhere.

Online blogs:

Reflections in a Head Mirror
https://www.froedtert.com/stories/reflections

A Fullness of Uncertain Significance
www.BruceCampbellMD.com

The Kern Institute *Transformational Times*
https://www.mcw.edu/departments/kern-institute/resources/
transformation-newsletters

Print / online publications:

A Piece of My Mind: The Book. Reproduced with permission from *JAMA: The Journal of the American Medical Association* 2007 (October 10); 298: 1613-1614. Copyright © 2007 American Medical Association. All rights reserved.

Auscult: Stories from Within (The Literary and Arts Journal of the Medical College of Wisconsin)

- The Transition, *Auscult* 2005
- Chocolate and Liquor, *Auscult* 2007
- Thank You for Calling Dr. Bob's Office, *Auscult* 2013
- I'm Ready, *Auscult* 2015

Acknowledgements

This is a book about my journey into and through medicine, so thanks, first and foremost, to the patients, families, physicians, residents, students, nurses, and hospital workers whose stories appear here. I am eternally grateful to each of you.

To my clinical colleagues at Froedtert Hospital, the Zablocki Veterans Affairs Medical Center, and the Medical College of Wisconsin, especially Becky Massey, Mike Stadler, Joe Zenga, Kathy Myers, Amanda Brandon, Rachel Stephenson, Chris Schultz, Michelle Michel, Stu Wong, and the late Robert Toohill, I am forever grateful for your partnership, guidance, and inspiration. I keep learning every day.

To my MCW colleagues who believe in the power of narrative, especially Art Derse and Adina Kalet, I admire your tireless efforts to expand the role of the medical humanities in health education.

To my American and African colleagues who share their treasure trove of stories, especially Susan and Kyle Cordes, Diana Sullivan, Henry Ngoitsi Nono, Titus Sisenda, Denge Makaya, and Owen Menach, I say *asante sana*.

To my classmates, teachers, and role models in the Narrative Medicine Program at Columbia University, especially Rita Charon and Cindy Smalletz, I say thanks for developing a wonderful curriculum and bringing science and rigor to narrative practice and medical training.

To my roundtable groups, especially Joanne Nelson, Aleta Chossek, Joel Habush, Pam Parker, Jennifer Rupp, and Myles Hopper at Red Oak Writing, and Dick Holloway, Nancy Havas, Tony Braza, Brittany Bettendorf, and K. Jane Lee in the MCW Moving Pens, I say thanks for sharing your work, for reading mine, and for pushing me.

To Kim Suhr, Director of Red Oak Writing, who acted as a role model, editor, cajoler, reviser, advisor, and voice asking, "Can you think of a better way to say that?" and "What does this seem to be about?" I am forever grateful. This book would never have made it to the finish line without you.

To the wonderful, enthusiastic team at Orange Hat Publishing/Ten16 Press, especially publisher Shannon Ishizaki, art director Kaeley Dunteman, illustrator Jayden Ellsworth, managing editor Lauren Blue, and my editor, Jenna Zerbel, I say thanks for your hard work, eye for quality, and professionalism at every point along the journey.

To my parents, Ray and Thora Campbell who were both gifted writers amidst all of the remarkable things they accomplished in their lives, I say thanks for passing along a love of endlessly rearranging words on a page. Rest in peace.

And, of course, to my sweet wife, Kathi, who makes it all possible, and to our children, Daniel, Sarah, David, and Rebekah, who bring joy, richness, delightful spouses/significant others, and now the next generation into our growing, story-enriched family, I love and cherish you all. You're the best!

About the Author

Bruce H. Campbell, MD FACS is a head and neck surgeon at the Medical College of Wisconsin (MCW).

He grew up in River Forest, Illinois and received a degree in biology from Purdue University in 1976. After graduating from Rush Medical College in 1980, he completed his otolaryngology residency at MCW in 1985, and a head and neck surgery fellowship at MD Anderson Cancer Center in 1987. He then returned to MCW, where he has spent his entire career. Because of his growing interest in the value of stories in healthcare, he earned a Certificate of Professional Achievement in Narrative Medicine from Columbia University in 2019.

Clinically, he has focused on seeing patients and performing surgery while engaging with medical students and residents. Throughout his career, he has also participated in clinical research, served in a variety of leadership roles, joined in global humanitarian work, and supported the development of the medical humanities.

He holds academic appointments in the MCW Department of Otolaryngology and Communication Sciences, the MCW Institute for Health and Equity (Bioethics and Medical Humanities), and the Robert D. and Patricia E. Kern Institute for the Transformation of Medical Education.

In addition to creative nonfiction, he has published humor,

poetry, and fiction. His work has appeared in a variety of medical and nonmedical journals including *JAMA: The Journal of the American Medical Association*, *Journal of Clinical Oncology*, *Creative Wisconsin*, *Narrative Inquiry in Bioethics*, and *The Examined Life Journal: A Literary Journal of the Carver College of Medicine*. Much of his writing is archived in his blog, *Reflections in a Head Mirror*, and at www.BruceCampbellMD.com.

He and his wife, Kathi, live near Milwaukee, WI.

Printed in the USA
CPSIA information can be obtained
at www.ICGtesting.com
LVHW071923200124
769493LV00014B/25/J